The
Hands-on Gui
to Data Interpretation

T0252447

SASHA ABRAHAM
GP Registrar
London Deanery
London, UK

KUNAL KULKARNI
Foundation Doctor
Oxford Deanery
Oxford, UK

RASHMI MADHU
GP Registrar
East Midlands Deanery
Nottingham, UK

DREW PROVAN
Senior Lecturer in Haematology
Academic Haematology Unit
Blizard Institute of Cell and Molecular Science
Barts and The London School of Medicine and Dentistry
Queen Mary University of London
London, UK

⊛WILEY-BLACKWELL
A John Wiley & Sons, Ltd., Publication

This edition first published 2010, © 2010 by S Abraham, K Kulkarni, R Madhu, D Provan

Blackwell Publishing was acquired by John Wiley & Sons in February 2007. Blackwell's publishing program has been merged with Wiley's global Scientific, Technical and Medical business to form Wiley-Blackwell.

Registered office: John Wiley & Sons Ltd, The Atrium, Southern Gate, Chichester, West Sussex PO19 8SQ, UK

Editorial offices: 9600 Garsington Road, Oxford OX4 2DQ, UK
                        The Atrium, Southern Gate, Chichester, West Sussex PO19 8SQ, UK
                        111 River Street, Hoboken, NJ 07030-5774, USA

For details of our global editorial offices, for customer services and for information about how to apply for permission to reuse the copyright material in this book please see our website at www.wiley.com/wiley-blackwell

Wiley also publishes its books in a variety of electronic formats. Some content that appears in print may not be available in electronic books.

Designations used by companies to distinguish their products are often claimed as trademarks. All brand names and product names used in this book are trade names, service marks, trademarks or registered trademarks of their respective owners. The publisher is not associated with any product or vendor mentioned in this book. This publication is designed to provide accurate and authoritative information in regard to the subject matter covered. It is sold on the understanding that the publisher is not engaged in rendering professional services. If professional advice or other expert assistance is required, the services of a competent professional should be sought.

Library of Congress Cataloging-in-Publication Data

The hands-on guide to data interpretation / Sasha Abraham ... [et al.].
    p. ; cm.
  Includes index.
  ISBN 978-1-4051-5256-3
1. Reference values (Medicine)–Handbooks, manuals, etc.   2. Diagnosis, Laboratory–Handbooks, manuals, etc. I. Abraham, Sasha.
    [DNLM: 1. Diagnostic Techniques and Procedures–Handbooks.   2. Laboratory Techniques and Procedures–Handbooks.   3. Medical Records–Handbooks.   WB 39 H23698 2010]
    RB38.2.H373 2010
    616.07'5–dc22

                                    2010015124

A catalogue record for this book is available from the British Library.

Set in 8 on 10 pt Humanist Light by Toppan Best-set Premedia Limited
Printed in Singapore

1   2010

Contents

Preface

There is no shortage of data – the attributes or measures assigned to a variable – in clinical medicine. With growth in both the number of available investigative modalities and the volume of investigations performed in clinical practice, the challenge of data interpretation lies in the translation of relevant raw data into information that can be appropriately applied to clinical decision making.

To condense the vast potential remit of this book, we have decided to focus on the interpretation of data derived from the more commonly encountered investigations in clinical practice. We have therefore attempted to limit the inclusion of approaches to interpreting data derived from other clinical activities such as clinical history taking and examination. However, this has not been an easy task (particularly in certain specialties, such as neurology), as these activities are – quite rightly – inextricably linked to the investigations performed as part of the management of patients. Notwithstanding the subject of this book, it is important to remember that the history and examination of patients remains at the core of patient management and investigations should be performed only as an adjunct to these processes – not as a replacement. Fundamentally, the interpretation of data derived from investigative procedures should always be undertaken with the clinical context in mind.

For medical students and junior doctors alike, data interpretation is a common feature of both examinations and clinical practice. This textbook aims to serve as an aide memoire, providing a concise repository of facts, figures and succinct explanations that can be used during both revision and clinical attachments. With the origins of this book stemming from our own clinical finals examination revision notes, each chapter has been written with close input from specialists in the field and highlights the approach to interpreting the key data sets encountered in a particular specialty. The 'patient data' chapter aims to bring all of these specialties together to consider some of the more practical aspects of interpreting and presenting data encountered in a clinical setting.

We hope that readers will find this textbook of use and that it will help put some structure to the multiple – and at times unwieldy – channels of data encountered in medical practice.

SA, KK, RM, DP

Acknowledgements

We would like to thank the following people for their help in the preparation of this book.

Sonya Abraham, Senior Lecturer in Rheumatology and Medicine, Kennedy Institute of Rheumatology, Imperial College Healthcare NHS Trust, London

Philip Bejon, Senior Research Fellow, Biomedical Research Centre, Oxford

Mark Blunden, Consultant Nephrologist, Barts and The London Hospitals, London

Anne Bolton, Head of Ophthalmic Imaging, Oxford Eye Hospital, Oxford

Muhammed Zameel Cader, Clinician Scientist and Honorary Consultant Neurologist, Oxford Centre for Gene Function, Oxford

Peter J Charles, Lead Biomedical Scientist, Translational Research, Kennedy Institute of Rheumatology, Imperial College, London

Fiona Cuthbertson, Specialist Registrar in Ophthalmology, Oxford Eye Hospital, Oxford

Andrew Davies, Senior Lecturer in Medical Oncology, and Honorary Consultant Cancer Sciences Division, University of Southampton School of Medicine, Southampton

Michelle Emery, Consultant in Endocrinology and Diabetes, Homerton University Hospital, London

Adrian Lim, Consultant Radiologist, Imperial College Healthcare NHS Trust, Hammersmith and Charing Cross Hospitals, London

Taya Kitiyakara, Consultant Gastroenterologist, Ramathibodi Hospital, Mahidol University, Bangkok, Thailand

George Markose, Consultant Radiologist, St George's Hospital, London

Peter Morgan-Warren, Specialty Registrar in Ophthalmology, West Midlands

Abdul Mozid, Cardiology Specialist Registrar, Essex Cardiothoracic Centre, Basildon

Geoffrey E Packe, Consultant Physician in Chest and General Medicine, Newham University Hospital, London

Zeudi Ramsey-Marcelle, ST7 Obstetrics and Gynaecology, North Middlesex University Hospital, London

Simon Richardson, Academic Clinical Fellow, Haemato-oncology, University College, London

Stefanie Christina Robert, Locum Consultant in Acute Medicine, Royal London Hospital, London

Sherif Sadek, Consultant Radiologist, Whipps Cross University Hospital, London

Parveen Vitish-Sharma, CT2 in General Surgery, St George's Hospital, London

Abbreviations

1/7	one day	ATN	acute tubular necrosis
1/12	one month	AV	atrioventricular
1/52	one week	AVPU	Alert, Voice, Pain, Unresponsive
18-FDG	18-fluorodeoxyglucose		
AIH1	autoimmune hepatitis 1	BC	bone conduction
AIH2	autoimmune hepatitis 2	Bd	bis in die (twice per day)
ABG	arterial blood gas	BE	base excess
ABP	arterial blood pressure	B-HCG	beta human chorionic gonadotrophin
ABPI	Ankle Brachial Pressure Index	BMI	body mass index
AC	air conduction	BPH	benign prostatic hyperplasia
ACE	angiotensin-converting enzyme	BS	bowel/breath sounds
ACS	acute coronary syndrome	BSEP	brainstem sensory evoked potential
ACTH	adrenocorticotrophic hormone	CABG	coronary artery bypass graft
ADH	antidiuretic hormone	CCP	cyclic citrullinated peptide
ADP	adenosine diphosphate	CEA	carcinoembryonic antigen
ADPKD	autosomal dominant polycystic kidney disease	CF	cystic fibrosis
AF	atrial fibrillation	CHD	coronary heart disease
AFP	alpha-fetoprotein	CJD	Creutzfeldt-Jakob disease
ALP	alkaline phosphatase	CK	creatine kinase
ALT	alanine aminotransferase	CLO	Campylobacter-like organism
AMA	anti-mitochondrial antibody	CMAP	compound muscle action potential
AML	acute myeloid leukaemia	CML	chronic myeloid leukaemia
ANA	anti-nuclear antibody	CMV	cytomegalovirus
ANCA	anti-neutrophil cytoplasmic antibody	CNS	central nervous system
		COPD	chronic obstructive pulmonary disease
APTT	activated partial thromboplastin time	COX	cyclooxygenase
ARDS	acute respiratory distress syndrome	CPET	cardiopulmonary exercise testing
ARPKD	autosomal recessive polycystic kidney disease	CRP	C-reactive protein
		CSF	cerebrospinal fluid
ASM	anti-smooth muscle antibody	CT	computed tomography
		CTG	cardiotocography
ASOT	anti-streptolysin O titre	CTPA	computed tomography pulmonary angiogram
AST	aspartate transaminase		

CTU	computed tomography urogram
CVA	cerebrovascular accident (stroke)
CVD	cardiovascular disease
CVP	central venous pressure
CXR/AXR	chest/abdominal X-ray
DI	diabetes insipidus
DIC	disseminated intravascular coagulation
DKA	diabetic ketoacidosis
DM	diabetes mellitus
DMSA	dimercaptosuccinic acid
DTPA	diethylene triamine penta-acetic acid
DVT	deep vein thrombosis
DWI	diffusion weighted imaging
ECG	electrocardiogram
ECT	electroconvulsive therapy
EEG	electroencephalogram
ELISA	enzyme-linked immunosorbent assay
EMG	electromyelogram
EOG	electrooculography
ERCP	endoscopic retrograde cholangio-pancreatograhy
ERV	expiratory reserve volume
ESR	erythrocyte sedimentation rate
ESWL	extracorporeal shock wave lithotripsy
FBC	full blood count
FDP	fibrin degradation product
FEV_1	forced expiratory volume (in 1 second)
FLAIR	fluid attenuated inversion recovery
FNA	fine needle aspiration
FOB	faecal occult blood
FRC	functional residual capacity
FSH	follicle-stimulating hormone
FVC	forced vital capacity
G6PD	glucose-6-phosphate dehydrogenase deficiency
GBS	Guillain-Barré syndrome

GCS	Glasgow Coma Scale
GFR	glomerular filtration rate
GGT	gamma glutamyl transferase
GH	growth hormone
GI	gastrointestinal
GORD	gastro-oesophageal reflux disease
Hb	haemoglobin
HBV	hepatitis B virus
HCC	hepatocellular carcinoma
hCG	human chorionic gonadotrophin
Hct	haematocrit
HDL	high density lipoprotein
HIFU	high intensity focused ultrasound
HLA	human leukocyte antigen
HMMA	hydroxymethylmandelic acid
HMPAO	hexamethylene propyleamine oxime
HONK	hyperosmolar non-ketotic
HR	heart rate
HSV	herpes simplex virus
HUS	haemolytic uraemic syndrome
IBD	inflammatory bowel disease
IC	inspiratory capacity
IGF-1	insulin-like growth factor
IHD	ischaemic heart disease
IM	intramuscularly
INR	international normalised ratio
IRV	inspiratory reserve volume
IU	international units
IV	intravenous
IVC	inferior vena cava
IVDU	intravenous drug use
IVP	intravenous pyelogram
IVU	intravenous urogram
JACCOL	jaundice/anaemia/cyanosis/ clubbing/oedema/ lymphadenopathy
JVP	jugular venous pressure
K_{CO}	carbon monoxide gas transfer coefficient

LAD	left axis deviation	NAC	N-acetylcysteine
LBBB	left bundle branch block	NAD	nothing abnormal detected
LDH	lactate dehydrogenase	NASH	non-alcoholic steato hepatitis
LDL	low density lipoprotein	NCS	nerve conduction studies
LFT	liver function test	NHL	non-Hodgkin's lymphoma
LH	luteinising hormone	NSAID	non-steroidal anti-inflammatory drug
LHRH	luteinising hormone-releasing hormone	OCP	ova, cysts, parasites
LFTs	liver function tests	OD	omni die (once per day)
LMN	lower motor neuron	OGD	oesophageal gastroduodenoscopy
LMWH	low-molecular weight heparin	PACS	picture archiving and communication system
LP	lumbar puncture	PAN	polyarteritis nodosa
L/RIF	left/right iliac fossa	PAPP-A	pregnancy associated plasma protein A
L/RUQ	left/right upper quadrant of the abdomen	P_aCO_2	partial pressure of carbon dioxide
L/RVF	left/right ventricular failure	P_aO_2	partial pressure of oxygen
LVH	left-ventricular hypertrophy	PBC	primary biliary cirrhosis
MAC	*Mycobacterium avium complex*	PCOS	polycystic ovarian syndrome
MCH	mean corpuscular haemoglobin	PCP	*Pneumocystis carinii* pneumonia
MCHC	mean cell haemoglobin concentration	PCR	polymerase chain reaction
MCUG	micturating cysturethrogram	PCV	packed cell volume
MCV	mean cell volume, mean corpuscular volume	PE	pulmonary embolus
		PEFR	peak expiratory flow rate
MEN	multiple endocrine neoplasia	PERLA	pupils equal and reactive to light and accommodation
MI	myocardial infarction		
MIBG	meta-iodo-benzyl-guanidine	PET	positron emission tomography
MMSE	mini-mental state examination	PKD	polycystic kidney disease; pyruvate kinase deficiency
MRA	magnetic resonance angiography	PL	prolactin
MRI	magnetic resonance imaging	PND	paroxysmal nocturnal dyspnoea
MRSA	methicillin-resistant *Staphylococcus aureus*	PNS	peripheral nervous system
MRV	magnetic resonance venography	PO	orally
		PR	per rectum, rectally
MS	multiple sclerosis	PRN	as required
MSU	mid-stream urine	PRV	polycythaemia rubra vera
NABQI	N-acetyl-p-benzoquinone imine	PSA	prostate specific antigen
		PSC	primary sclerosing cholangitis

PT	prothrombin time	SVT	supraventricular tachycardia
PTC	percutaneous trans-hepatic cholangiography	T3	tri-iodo
		T4	thyroxine
PTH	parathyroid hormone	TB	tuberculosis
PUBS	percutaneous umbilical cord blood sampling	TBG	thyroxine-binding globulin
		TDS	ter die sumendus (three times per day)
PUO	pyrexia of unknown origin		
QDS	quater die sumendus (four times per day)	TFTS	thyroid function tests
		TIA	transient ischaemic attack
RA	rheumatoid arthritis	TIBC	total iron-binding capacity
RBBB	right bundle branch block	TLC	total lung capacity
RBC	red blood cell	TOE	transoesophageal echo
RF	risk factor, rheumatoid factor	TRH	thyrotrophin-releasing hormone
RIBA	radioimmunoblot assay	TRUS	transrectal ultrasound
RR	respiration rate	TSH	thyroid stimulating hormone
RTA	renal tubular acidosis	TT	thrombin time
rt-PA	recombinant tissue-plasminogen activator	TTE	transthoracic echocardiography
RV	residual volume	tTG	tissue transglutaminase
SA	sinoatrial	TTP	thrombotic thrombocytopenic purpura
SAH	subarachnoid haemorrhage		
SBP	spontaneous bacterial peritonitis	TV	tidal volume
		U&E	urea and electrolytes
S/C	subcutaneous	UC	ulcerative colitis
SEP	sensory evoked potential	UMN	upper motor neuron
SHBG	sex hormone binding globulin	US	ultrasound
		UTI	urinary tract infection
SIRS	systemic inflammatory response syndrome	VC	vital capacity
		VEP	visual evoked potential
SLA	soluble liver antigen	VF	ventricular fibrillation
SLE	systemic lupus erythematosus	VMA	vanillylmandelic acid
		VT	ventricular tachycardia
SOB(OE)	shortness of breath (on exertion)	VTE	venous thromboembolism
		WCC	white cell count
SPECT	single photon emission computed tomography	WHO	World Health Organization
		WPW	Wolff-Parkinson-White
STIR	short tau inversion recovery	ZN	Ziehl-Neelsen
SVC	superior vena cava		

Chapter 1
NORMAL RANGES

Notes

1 All are serum values (unless otherwise stated).

2 'Normal range' values differ between individual laboratories and normal healthy individuals, as well as different ages and sexes. Furthermore, disease processes beyond those commonly associated with a particular 'abnormality' may be associated with variations in individual measurements.

For example, elevated ESR levels may be found in heart failure (even in the absence of the presence of any of the common 'normal' causes of elevated ESR). Quoted reference intervals should therefore be considered as guides rather than absolute values, and should always be considered in the clinical context.

3 All values are for adults unless otherwise stated.

Haematology

Full blood count (FBC)

Haemoglobin (Hb)		13.0–18.0 g/dL (males), 11.5–16.5 g/dL (females)
Mean cellular volume (MCV)		80–96 fL
Packed cell volume (PCV)/Haematocrit (Hct)		40–50% (males), 36–45% (females)
Mean corpuscular haemoglobin (MCH)		28–32 pg
Mean cell haemoglobin concentration (MCHC)		32–35 g/dL
Reticulocytes		$25–85 \times 10^9$/L or 0.5–2.4%
Platelets		$150–400 \times 10^9$/L
White cell count (WCC)		$4–11 \times 10^9$/L
Differential WCC:	Neutrophils	$2.5–7.5 \times 10^9$/L
	Lymphocytes	$1.5–4.0 \times 10^9$/L
	Monocytes	$0.2–0.8 \times 10^9$/L
	Eosinophils	$0.04–0.44 \times 10^9$/L
	Basophils	$0.0–0.1 \times 10^9$/L

The hands-on guide to data interpretation. By S. Abraham, K. Kulkarni, R. Madhu and D. Provan. Published 2010 by Blackwell Publishing Ltd.

Others

Erythrocyte sedimentation rate (ESR)	0–15 mm/1st hour (males), 0–30 mm/1st hour (females)

Coagulation screen

Prothrombin time (PT)	12–15 s
Activated partial thromboplastin time (APTT)	40–50 s
Bleeding time	3–8 min
International normalised ratio (INR)	<0.9–1.2
Fibrinogen	1.8–5.4 g/L
D-Dimer	<0.5 mg/L (varies with assay used, e.g. ELISA/latex agglutination, etc.)

Haematinics

Iron	12–30 µmol/L
Total iron-binding capacity (TIBC)	45–75 µmol/L
Ferritin	15–300 µg/L
Transferrin	2.0–4.0 g/L
B12	160–760 ng/L
Folate	2.0–11.0 µg/L
Red cell folate	160–640 µg/L
Haptoglobins	0.13–1.63 g/L

Haemoglobin electrophoresis (normal adults)

Haemoglobin A	>95%
Haemoglobin A2	2–3%
Haemoglobin F	<2%

Chemistry

Ions	
Sodium (Na$^+$)	137–144 mmol/L
Potassium (K$^+$)	3.5–5.0 mmol/L
Chloride (Cl$^-$)	95–107 mmol/L
Bicarbonate (HCO$_3^-$)	20–28 mmol/L
Corrected calcium (Ca^{2+})	2.2–2.6 mmol/L
Phosphate (PO^{4+})	0.8–1.4 mmol/L
Copper (Cu^{2+})	12–26 µmol/L
Caeruloplasmin	200–350 mg/L
Magnesium (Mg^{2+})	0.75–1.05 mmol/L
Anion gap	12–16 mmol/L
	Calculated by: $([Na^+]+[K^+])-([Cl^-]+[HCO_3^-])$
Renal	
Urea	2.5–7.5 mmol/L
Creatinine	60–110 µmol/L
Urate	0.23–0.46 mmol/L (males), 0.19–0.36 mmol/L (females)
Plasma osmolality	278–305 mosmol/kg

(Continued)

(Continued)

Hepatic	
Total protein	61–76 g/L
Albumin	37–49 g/L
Total bilirubin	1–22 µmol/L
Conjugated bilirubin	0–3.4 µmol/L
Alanine aminotransferase (ALT)	5–35 U/L
Aspartate aminotransferase (AST)	1–31 U/L
Alkaline phosphatase (ALP)	45–105 U/L (over 14 years)
Gamma glutamyl transferase (GGT)	4–35 U/L (<50 U/L in males)
Lactate dehydrogenase (LDH)	10–250 U/L

Cardiac	
Creatine kinase MB fraction	<5%
Troponin I	0–0.4 µg/L
Troponin T	0–0.1 µg/L

Others	
Creatine kinase (CK)	24–195 U/L (males), 24–170 U/L (females)
Plasma lactate	0.6–1.8 mmol/L
Fasting plasma glucose	3.0–6.0 mmol/L
Haemoglobin A1 C (HbA₁C)	3.8–6.4%
Fructosamine	<285 µmo/L
Serum amylase	60–180 U/L

Lipids and lipoproteins

NB: These target levels vary depending on the patient's overall cardiovascular risk assessment.

Cholesterol	<5.2 mmol/L
LDL (low density lipoprotein) cholesterol	<3.36 mmol/L
HDL (high density lipoprotein) cholesterol	>1.55 mmol/L
Fasting serum triglyceride	0.45–1.69 mmol/L

Blood gases

(See Chapter 3 for further information)

H⁺	35–45 nmol/L
pH	7.35–7.45
PaO₂	10.6–12.6 kPa
PaCO₂	4.7–6.0 kPa
Base excess	±2 mmol/L

NB: 1 kPa = 7.6 mmHg. Atmospheric pressure approximately 100 kPa.

Hormones

Adrenal

Serum aldosterone (normal diet)	Upright (4h): 330–830 pmol/L Supine (30 min): 135–400 pmol/L
Serum cortisol	09.00: 200–700 nmol/L 22.00: 50–200 nmol/L
Urinary cortisol	<280 nmol/24 h

Dexamethasone suppression test	Overnight (after 1 mg dexamethasone):
	   cortisol <50 nmol/l
	Low dose test (2 mg/day for 48 h):
	   cortisol <50 nmol/L

Serum oestradiol
   Males
   Females
	
	<180 pmol/L
	Post-menopausal: <100 pmol/L
	Follicular: 200–400 pmol/L
	Mid-cycle: 400–1200 pmol/L
	Luteal: 400–1000 pmol/L

Serum progesterone
   Males (very rarely undertaken)
   Females:
	
	<6 nmol/L
	Follicular <10 nmol/L
	Luteal >30 nmol/L (should be checked
	   on day 21 of 28-day menstrual cycle)

Serum testosterone
   Males
   Females
	
	9–35 nmol/L
	0.5–3 nmol/L

Anterior pituitary

Plasma adrenocorticotrophic hormone (ACTH)	09.00: <18 pmol/L

Plasma follicle stimulating
hormone (FSH)
   Males
   Females
	
	1–7 U/L
	Follicular: 2.5–10 U/L
	Mid-cycle: 25–70 U/L
	Luteal: 0.32–2.1 U/L
	Post-menopausal: >30 U/L

Plasma growth hormone (GH)
   Basal, fasting and between
pulses:
   After hypoglycaemia
	
	<1 mU/L
	
	>40 mU/L (many centres accept values
	>20 mU/L)

(Continued)

(Continued)

Plasma luteinising hormone (LH)	
Males	1–10 U/L
Females	Follicular: 2.5–10 U/L
	Mid-cycle: 25–70 U/L
	Luteal: 1–13 U/L
	Post-menopausal: >30 U/L
Plasma prolactin (PL)	65–490 mIU/L (females), 55–340 mIU/L (males) *or* 1–25 ng/mL (females), 1–20 ng/mL (males)

Posterior pituitary

Plasma antidiuretic hormone (ADH)	0.9–4.6 pmol/L (NB: random values can be meaningless – need to measure this in the context of hydration status and should ideally be measured only in the specialist context of a controlled hypertonic saline infusion test)

Thyroid

Plasma thyroid binding globulin (TBG)	13–28 mg/L (not routinely measured in clinical practice)
Plasma thyroid stimulating hormone (TSH)	0.4–5 mU/L
Total plasma thyroxine (T4)	58–174 nmol/L
Free T4	10–22 pmol/L
Total tri-iodothyronine (T3)	1.07–3.18 nmol/L
Free T3	5–10 pmol/L
Serum TSH receptor antibodies	<7 U/L
Serum antithyroid peroxidase	<50 IU/mL

Others

Plasma parathyroid hormone (PTH)	0.9–5.4 pmol/L
Plasma calcitonin	<27 pmol/L (should be measured in fasting state)
Serum cholecalciferol (vitamin D3)	60–105 nmol/L
Serum 25-OH-cholecalciferol	45–90 nmol/L

Tumour markers

NB: These values can be meaningless when interpreted outside the appropriate clinical context. Tumour markers are best used for monitoring treatment response and tumour recurrence, as well as for diagnosis when considered alongside relevant clinical and other investigative findings.

Alpha-fetoprotein (AFP)	<10 kU/L
Carcinoembryonic antigen (CEA)	<10 µg/L
Neurone specific enolase	<12 µg/L
Prostate specific antigen (PSA)	<4 µg/L (males >40 years) / <2 µg/L (males <40 years)
Human chorionic gonadotrophin (B-HCG)	<5 U/L
CA 125	<35 U/mL
CA 19-9	<33 U/mL

Cerebrospinal fluid

Opening pressure	50–200 mm H_2O
Protein	0.15–0.45 g/L
Albumin	0.066–0.442 g/L
Chloride	116–122 mmol/L
Glucose	2.2–4.4 mmol/L (>50% plasma glucose)
Lactate	1–2 mmol/L
Red cell count	0/mm³
White cell count	≤5/mm³
Differential	
Lymphocytes	60–70% (<5/mm³)
Monocytes	30–50%
Neutrophils	None

Sweat

| Chloride | 60 mmol/L (higher values are consistent with a diagnosis of cystic fibrosis) *NB:* Some sources use higher values for the diagnosis of CF |

Immunoglobulins

IgM	0.45–2.0 g/L
IgG	7.0–14.5 g/L
IgA	0.8–4.0 g/L

Urine

Glomerular filtration rate (GFR)	70–140 mL/min
Creatinine clearance (an estimate of GFR)	75–115 mL/min (females), 82–125 mL/min (males)
Total protein	<150 mg/24 h
Albumin	<30 mg/24 h
Albumin/creatinine ratio	<3.5 mg/mmol (males), <2.5 mg/mmol (females)
Sodium	100–250 mmol/24 h
Potassium	14–120 mmol/24 h
Phosphate (inorganic)	15–50 mmol/24 h
Calcium	2.5–7.5 mmol/24 h
Urobilinogen	1.7–5.9 μmol/24 h
Osmolality	350–1000 mosmol/kg
5-HT metabolite 5-Hydroxyindole acetic acid (HIAA)	16–73 μmol/24 h
Catecholamine and metabolites Noradrenaline Adrenaline Metanephrines	60–660 nmol/24 h 15–160 nmol/24 h 0.03–0.695 μmol/mmol creatinine or <5.5 μmol/24 h
Hydroxymethylmandelic acid (HMMA)/ vanillylmandelic acid (VMA)	16–48 μmol/24 h

NB: Most centres are moving away from the measurement of VMA due to its poor relative sensitivity as compared to catecholamines and metanephrines.

Units and conversion tables

■ Always write out the abbreviation in full when documenting in notes or charts (especially drug prescription charts) – for example, write 'milligrams' rather than 'mg') to avoid confusion.

■ Errors cost lives: a slight misinterpretation of what unit is written (for example, if 'μg' looks like 'mg') could lead to a 1,000-fold increase in the dose administered. These errors happen but can be prevented.

Length

1 centimetre (cm)	10 millimetres (mm)
1 metre (m)	100 centimetres (cm) = 1000 millimetres (mm)
1 inch	25.4 millimetres (mm)
1 foot	12 inches = 304.8 millimetres (cm)

Mass

1 nanogram (ng)	1000 picograms (pg)
1 microgram (μg)	1000 nanograms (ng)
1 milligram (mg)	1000 micrograms (μg)
1 gram (g)	1000 milligrams (mg)
1 kilogram (kg)	1000 grams (g)
1 pound (lb)	0.45 kilograms (kg)

Volume

1 millilitre (mL)	1000 microlitres (μL)
1 litre (L)	1000 millilitres (mL)
1 pint	Approximately 568 mL
1 decilitre (dL)	100 millilitres (mL)
1 fluid ounce (fl oz)	Approximately 29.6 mL
1 unit per litre (U/L)	Also written as IU/L (international units/litre)
milliunits per litre (mU/L)	10^{-3} units/litre
kilounits pre litre (kU/L)	10^3 units/litre

Concentration

mole (mol)	SI base unit of the amount of a substance – amount of substance of a system that contains an equivalent number of elementary entities (e.g. atoms, molecules, electrons, etc.) as there are atoms in 12 g of carbon-12 (^{12}C)
millimole (mmol)	10^{-3} mol
micromole (μmol)	10^{-6} mol
picomole (pmol)	10^{-12} mol
osmole (osmol)	1 osmole is one gram molecular weight (1 mole) of any non-dissociable substance, and contains 6.02×10^{23} particles
milliosmole (mosmol)	10^{-3} osmol

Pressure

pascal (Pa)	measure of force per unit area (one newton per square metre)
kilopascal	1000 Pa

Chapter 2
CARDIOVASCULAR

Introduction

This chapter will focus on some of the practical applications of cardiac investigations. The electrocardiogram (ECG) is one of the commonest investigations that students and junior trainees encounter – and also one of the commonest investigations to cause panic. In this chapter, we have attempted to summarise the key facts about ECG interpretation to help refresh your memory as you practise. In addition, this chapter also discusses a number of other cardiovascular pathologies encountered on the wards, especially those diagnosed using blood tests – from enzymatic markers of ischaemic damage to the diagnostic interpretation of infective endocarditis and the immune phenomenon of rheumatic fever. Finally, we take a look at some physiology. In particular, we will consider the pressures and waveforms associated with the cardiac cycle and the jugular venous pressure (JVP) – both of which are common topics asked about on the ward.

Topics covered
- Electrocardiogram (ECG) interpretation
- Exercise tolerance test
- Cardiac enzymes
- Infective endocarditis

- Rheumatic fever
- Pressures and sounds
- Other cardiac investigations (e.g. echocardiography, coronary artery catheterisation)
- Peripheral vascular disease

Electrocardiogram (ECG) interpretation

Introduction

ECGs are comprised of multiple leads. These are recordings from different electrodes, each of which 'see' the heart from a different angle. While 3-lead ECGs are often found on emergency equipment (such as defibrillators), the 12-lead ECG is more commonly encountered. The leads of a 12-lead ECG comprise six chest leads (V1–6), the limb leads (I, II, III) and the augmented limb leads (aVL, aVR, aVF). These look at the following areas of the heart:

- **II, III, aVF:** inferior surface
- **aVR:** right side (right atrium)
- **V2-4:** left ventricular anterior wall and interventricular septum
- **V5-6, aVL, I:** lateral surface (left ventricle).

The hands-on guide to data interpretation. By S. Abraham, K. Kulkarni, R. Madhu and D. Provan. Published 2010 by Blackwell Publishing Ltd.

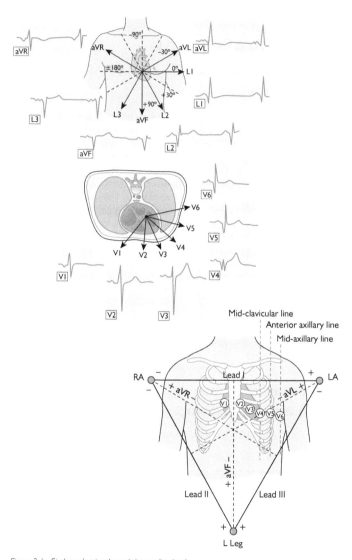

Figure 2.1: Einthoven's triangle and the cardiac leads

The normal ECG waveform

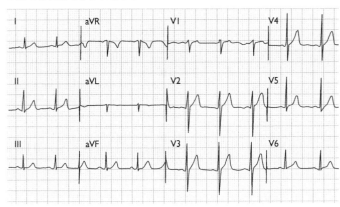

Figure 2.2: A normal ECG

Average time (whole cycle)	0.8 s
Standard machine speed	25 mm/s (10 mm = 1 mV)
1 small square (1 mm)	0.04 s (40 ms)
1 big square (5 mm)	0.2 s (200 ms)

NB: Rates given as beats per minute (bpm)

- P wave = atrial depolarisation (NB: atrial repolarisation cannot be seen as it occurs 'behind' the QRS complex).
- QRS complex (grouping of the Q, R and S waves) = ventricular depolarisation:
- Q = 1st downwards deflection after P wave
- R = 1st upwards deflection after P wave
- S = downwards deflection following R wave.
- T = ventricular repolarisation.

How to interpret ECGs

The key to understanding ECGs is to start at the beginning and work through the same sequence of interpretation every time. Always interpret

Five key basic items to consider
1. Check the details
2. Rate
3. Rhythm
4. Axis
5. Intervals and durations

Five important categories of abnormalities to consider
1. 1st, 2nd and 3rd degree heart block
2. Bundle branch blocks
3. Other blocks
4. Arrhythmias
5. Other abnormalities

ECGs in the clinical context of the patient, and remember to treat the patient not the tracing. A word of warning – do not always believe the machine interpretations given on the top of most ECGs.

The 10-step ECG interpretation guide

We will now consider the above 10 points in more detail.

1 Check the details
■ Patient details (name/date of birth/ hospital number).
■ Date and time of the tracing.
■ Any symptoms recorded as being present (e.g. chest pain).

■ If available, always compare the ECG with old tracings to look for changes.

2 Rate
■ ECG trace paper runs through the machine at 25 mm/s.
■ Ventricular rate = 300 divided by the number of big squares between successive R waves, e.g. if the R–R interval is 5 squares, then the rate is 300 divided by 5 = 60 bpm.
■ Atrial rate = as above, using the number of squares between successive P waves.
■ Usually, ventricular bradycardia means <60 bpm, tachycardia means >100 bpm. There are exceptions to this (e.g. a trained athlete may have a 'normal' resting heart rate of 40 bpm).

Squares:	1	2	3	4	5	6
Rate (bpm):	300	150	100	75	60	50

3 Rhythm

✓ **TIP:** Use the edge of a piece of paper held over the rhythm strip (usually lead II) to make markings for a few successive P waves (atrial rhythm) or R waves (ventricular rhythm). Then slide the paper along to see if the markings 'match up' with later portions of the tracing. This can help identify more subtle irregular rhythms.

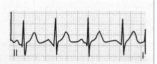

Figure 2.3: Determining the regularity of the rhythm

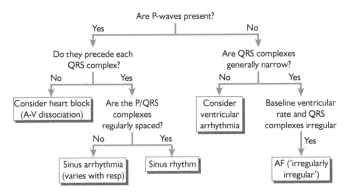

Figure 2.4: Approach to assessing the rhythm

REMEMBER:
- **narrow** complex = **atrial** origin
- **broad** complex = **ventricular** origin.

4 Axis
Estimating
The easiest way of estimating the axis is to use the following system.
- Right axis deviation: lead I QRS deflection primarily downwards (S>R)/ leads II and III upwards.
- Common causes: RVH, PE, antero-lateral MI.
- Left axis deviation: leads II and III QRS deflection primarily downwards/ lead I upwards.
- Common causes: left anterior fascicle block (left anterior hemiblock), inferior MI (ischaemic heart disease).
- See the 'heart block' and 'other blocks' sections for more information on conduction block.

Precise calculation
To calculate the axis more precisely, use the following method.

- Look at the R and S waves of leads I and aVF on the 12-lead ECG.
- Determine the approximate direction (up or down) and amount (number of squares) of overall deflection. For example:
  - lead I: R wave (upwards deflection) of 5 small squares and S wave (downwards deflection) of 1 small square, overall deflection = 4 small squares upwards
  - lead aVF: R wave (upwards deflection) of 2 small squares and S wave (downwards deflection) of 8 small square, overall deflection = 6 small squares downwards.
- Using the rule: overall upwards deflection = positive, overall downwards deflection = negative. Plot these approximate values along the axis chart to determine the axis.
  - The cardiac axis
    NB: arrows point towards positive.
    In this example, there is left axis deviation of approximately 55°. Note that the '180' on the right side of the arrow in both diagrams is not clearly visible.

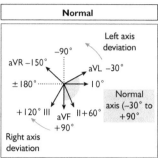

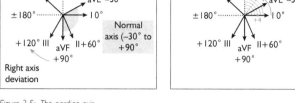

Figure 2.5: The cardiac axis

5 Intervals and durations

Normal (reference ranges)
PR interval (AV node delay)	= 200 ms (5 small squares)
QRS complex width (ventricular depolarisation)	= 120 ms (3 small squares)
QT interval (mechanical ventricular contraction)	= 400 ms (10 small squares)

■ Prolonged PR: 1st degree heart block.

■ Shortened PR: Wolff-Parkinson-White (WPW) syndrome.

■ Prolonged QT: electrolyte abnormality (hypocalcaemia, hypomagnesaemia, hypokalaemia), congenital syndromes (e.g. Romano-Ward, Jervell and Lang-Nielsen), drugs (e.g. amiodarone, sotalol, erythromycin) – increased risk of progression to *Torsades de Pointes*, hypothermia, acute myocardial ischaemia.

NB: The QT interval varies with heart rate and this is corrected for using the following calculation:

$$QTc = \frac{QT}{\sqrt{RR}}$$

Normal range for QTc: <450 ms (males), <470 ms (females)

6 Heart block

This is the failure or interruption of the normal flow of the electrical impulse through the heart. Aside from skipped beats/pauses, there are three main types.

■ Skipped beats/pauses: sinoatrial (SA) node failure to conduct so no P wave/QRS (not necessarily pathological).

■ 1st degree block: PR interval consistently prolonged. Can be seen in normal people (e.g. athletes) or in acute infarction/rheumatic fever.

■ 2nd degree block:

• Mobitz Type I – (Wenckebach type): progressively lengthening PR interval, eventually leading to a P wave that is not followed by a QRS complex

• 2nd degree block (Mobitz Type 2): occasional P-waves without a following QRS complex

–2nd degree block (2:1): this is a subset of Mobitz type 2 block. Two P waves preceding each QRS (similarly, 3:1 block is 3 P waves). 2nd degree blocks are often seen in more acute ischaemic situations.

■ 3rd degree block (complete heart block): no atrial contractions conducted to ventricles, so no relationship between P waves and QRS complexes (subsequently develop a regular slow 'escape' ventricular rhythm). Often due to fibrosis of the conducting system.

Pacing indications

Aside from any associated symptoms the patient may have, the danger with heart block is the risk of progression. 1st degree block usually only requires pacing for symptoms, i.e. secondary to bradycardia (especially if rate <40 bpm), syncope or if there are prolonged asystolic pauses (>3 s). Mobitz Type 2/2:1 block can progress to 3rd degree block, and so pacing is usually advised, particularly if it is associated with symptomatic bradycardia or asymptomatic patients with asystole >3 s or heart rate <40 bpm in awake patients. Contrary to previous practice, pacing should be considered for Wenckebach's, particularly in symptomatic patients complaining of pre-syncope/syncope, due to the risk of progression. 3rd degree block requires pacing as this can progress to ventricular tachycardia/ventricular fibrillation (VT/VF). Complete heart block is associated with 50% mortality at 1 year if left untreated.

Pacemaker types

Nomenclature follows the following pattern.

■ 'ABC': where A = chamber paced, B = chamber sensed and C = response.

■ Characters used: 0 = none, A = atrium, V = ventricle, D = dual, T = triggered, I = inhibited, R = rate modulated.

For example, a VVI pacemaker (**V**entricle sensed, **V**entricle paced, **I**nhibited by ventricular event) both senses and paces the ventricle and has an inhibitory response. Inhibitory means that a pacemaker does not actually 'kick in' if it senses an intrinsic heart beat, and as long as the intrinsic heart rate is above 60 bpm. This saves battery life and prevents patients from becoming pacemaker dependent.

The general rule is that patients in atrial flutter/fibrillation who require a pacemaker are fitted with a single-chamber PPM (permanent pacemaker, often a VVI), and patients who still have P waves on the ECG (e.g. in higher degree AV blocks) are fitted with a dual chamber pacemaker, which is normally programmed to DDD mode.

In a single chamber PPM, the lead is situated in the right ventricle, and in a dual chamber PPM, one lead is placed in the right atrium and the other one in the right ventricle.

7 Bundle branch block (BBB)

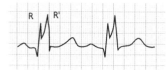

Figure 2.6: Left bundle branch block

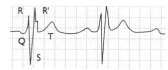

Figure 2.7: Right bundle branch block

■ Left BBB: 'WiLLiaM' (QRS complex in V1 = 'W' shaped, in V6 = 'M' shaped).
• Axis is either normal or left axis deviation.
• Note that it can be difficult to interpret more of the ECG if LBBB is present. However, it can still be possible to diagnose acute myocardial ischaemia by the presence of ST segment deviation (e.g. using the Sgarbossa criteria, although their sensitivity is low and their unsupervised use is not recommended).
■ Right BBB: 'MarRoW' (QRS complex in V1 = 'M' shaped (RSR¹ pattern), in V6 = 'W' shaped).
• Axis usually remains normal.

8 Other blocks

■ Bifascicular block: RBBB with left anterior fascicular block (left axis deviation, LAD) or RBBB with left posterior hemiblock.
■ Left anterior fascicular block (= left anterior hemiblock): positive QRS in lead I and negative QRS in aVF.
■ Left posterior hemiblock: this is much rarer. Features right axis deviation (RAD), with no evidence of right ventricular hypertrophy (RVH) or anterior infarction.
■ Trifascicular block: bifascicular block with 1st degree heart block. Note that alternating RBBB and LBBB are a sign of trifascicular block.
■ AV nodal block: the maximum AV nodal rate is 200/min, therefore at rates >200/min, AV block is possible. This is identified by some P waves having no QRS following them. In this scenario, the

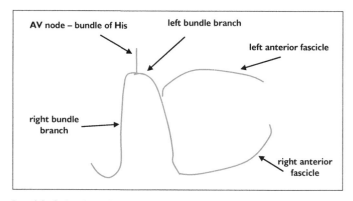

Figure 2.8: Cardiac electrical conduction pathways

AV node is still working (to slow A-V conduction), and the ventricular rate usually remains relatively normal.

9 Arrhythmias

Extrasystoles/escape rhythm

■ Narrow complex = supraventricular origin, wide complex = ventricular origin.

■ If of a junctional (around AV node) or a ventricular origin, then no P wave precedes the QRS.

■ If persistent, can suggest an 'escape' rhythm, a compensatory rhythm caused by a pacemaker at a site other than the normal SA/AV-nodal system.

Sinus arrhythmia

■ Normal variation in rate with respiration. Increased rate with inspiration.

Atrial fibrillation (AF)

■ 'Irregularly irregular' – no obvious P waves, narrow QRS complexes.

■ Causes of AF include:

• cardiac: ischaemic heart disease (IHD), hypertension, valvular disease (e.g. mitral valve)

• respiratory: infections (e.g. pneumonia), malignancy, pleural effusion

• endocrine disorders: e.g. thyrotoxicosis

• other: acute infection/sepsis, alcohol excess, post-operative.

■ Management: rate or rhythm control, decision on adequate stroke (embolic) prophylaxis (i.e. either antiplatelets or warfarin).

■ AF with BBB can resemble a broad-complex tachycardia.

Atrial flutter

■ Characteristic 'sawtooth' baseline, often at ventricular rates that are multiples of 150 (the atrial rate is usually >250/min).

■ Count the number of P waves preceding each QRS to determine type of block (2:1, etc.).

Supraventricular tachycardia (SVT)

■ Ventricular rate usually >150/min.

■ Narrow QRS complexes identify this as a supraventricular source (rather than ventricular).

■ If the source is near the AV node ('nodal' tachycardia), then no P waves are seen.

Ventricular tachycardia (VT)

■ Ventricular rate >120/min.

■ Every broad-complex tachycardia is VT unless proven otherwise.

■ Can be 'monophasic' (waveform is same amplitude throughout) or 'polymorphic' (differing amplitude waveforms).

■ Suggests a ventricular focus or source with abnormal conduction through the ventricle (hence wide).

■ Differential diagnosis: accelerated idioventricular rhythm (a prolonged ventricular focus 'escape' rhythm with rates greater than those seen in complete heart block – associated with acute MI), AF with conduction block.

Torsades de Pointes

■ Variant of VT with a 'twisting' pattern (varying morphology of QRS complexes around the isoelectric axis).

■ Usually occurs in 'bursts', associated with long-QT states.

■ Commonly associated with hypomagnesaemia so intravenous magnesium sulphate (2 g) should be administered.

Ventricular fibrillation (VF)

■ Disorganised tracing, no QRS complex identifiable, patient unconscious.
■ Caused by inefficient and inadequate contraction of ventricular muscle. Not compatible with any cardiac output.

Asystole

■ Very rarely a completely flat tracing.
■ Always check the leads and the gain on the ECG machine.

10 Other abnormalities
ST-segment changes

■ Elevation: can be normal ('high take-off'), acute MI, acute pericarditis ('saddle' shaped).
■ Depression: can be normal (upward sloping), digoxin (downward sloping), ischaemic (flat), posterior MI – changes in the posterior heart are seen as 'reciprocal' or 'reflected' changes (ST depression in leads V1–3).

T-wave changes

■ Peaking: hyperkalaemia, acute MI.
■ Inversion: V1–3 can be inverted in children/Afro-Caribbean people (normal), post acute-phase of MI, myocardial ischaemia and left-ventricular hypertrophy (LVH).

Drugs/electrolyte imbalance

■ Digoxin: 'reverse-tick' ST-segment (slopes downwards).
■ Hyperkalaemia: peaked/tented T waves, flattened P wave and ST segment, QRS complex widening, 'sine wave'-shaped ECG.
■ Hypokalaemia: 'U waves' (hump at end of T wave), flattened T waves, prolonged QT interval.

■ Hypocalcaemia: QT-interval prolongation (reverse in hypercalcaemia).

Myocardial hypertrophy

■ Left atrial hypertrophy: 'bifid' P waves (P mitrale).
■ Right atrial hypertrophy: peaked P waves (P ulmonale = eaked P waves).
■ Left ventricular hypertrophy: 'voltage criteria = R waves in V5/6 >25 mm or R wave in V5/6 + S wave in V1/2 >35 mm, Sokolov-Lyon index: sum of S in V1 and R in V5 or V6 > 35 mm, occasionally inverted T waves in I, aVL, V4/5/.
■ Right ventricular hypertrophy: tall R waves in V1 > 7 mm, R in V1 and S in V5 or V6 > 10 mm, T-wave inversion in V1/2 (sometimes in V3/4), deep S wave in V6, right axis deviation, occasionally RBBB.

Ischaemia/Myocardial infarction

■ ST-segment depression suggests ischaemia (although consider posterior infarction).
■ MI progression: peaked 'tombstone' T waves → ST-segment elevation → Q waves (sharp downwards slope >1 mm before QRS complex) → normalising ST segment → T-wave inversion.
■ Anterior infarction: V2–3.
■ Septal infarction: V3–4.
■ Inferior infarction: II, III and aVF.
■ Lateral infarction: I, aVL, V5–6.
■ Posterior infarction: dominant R waves in V1 (with 'ischaemic'-like ST-depression changes in other leads).

Pulmonary embolism

■ Usually see sinus tachycardia.
■ Classical ECG signs: S1-Q3-T3 (prominent S wave in I (right axis devia-

tion), Q waves and inverted T waves in lead III, this is a rare sign and predominantly occurs in patients who have a massive pulmonary embolus (PE).

■ Occasionally associated with right axis deviation (right heart strain), RBBB, dominant R wave in V1, inverted T waves in V1–3.

Pericarditis

■ 'Saddle'-shaped ST segments, usually throughout the ECG.

Wolff-Parkinson-White (WPW) syndrome

■ Accessory A-V conduction pathway (bundle of Kent) that bypasses AV node.

■ δ-wave: due to earlier partial ventricular depolarisation ('pre-excitation').

■ Symptoms: asymptomatic, chest discomfort/palpitations (due to paroxysmal narrow complex tachycardia that can be sustained due to an active 're-entry' circuit), dizziness, collapse (cardiac arrest). Often presents in teenagers/young adults.

■ Risks: can progress to VF, so can be treat by radiofrequency ablation.

Ambulatory (24-hour) ECG

■ This is also known as Holter monitoring.

■ 3–4 leads are usually used. These are attached to a recording box that is worn by the patient. The tracings can then be analysed to look for ECG changes that coincide with occurrence of the symptoms. On some machines, patients can press a button to mark when symptoms occur. With other recorders, patients keep a diary to record that time at which symptoms occur.

■ Ambulatory ECG recording is a helpful in investigating certain symptoms, particularly those that occur infrequently and unpredictably (e.g. syncope/dizziness, palpitations). There are three main types of recorders.

• Continuous rhythm recorders: these record all heart rhythm over a specified period of time, e.g. 24 or 48h. This is useful to detect diurnal heart rhythm changes but can be time-consuming to analyse.

• Event recorders: these are programmed to store heart rates above and below certain parameters (e.g. below 40bpm and above 120bpm) and are usually worn for 4–7 days.

• Implantable loop recorders (e.g. Memo or Reveal device): these are useful in patients who have infrequent symptoms. A small recording device is implanted in the subcutaneous tissue above the heart. The patient can activate the recorder when an event (e.g. syncope) is anticipated, by placing an activator over the device. The device stores a recording of the cardiac rhythm during and around the event, and can be left in place for a number of months.

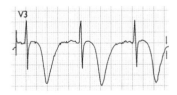

Figure 2.9: T-wave inversion and ST-depression (changes suggestive of ischaemia)

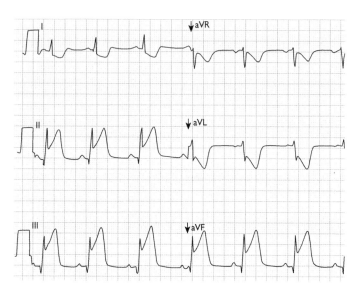

Figure 2.10: Inferior MI – ST-elevation in the inferior leads (II, III and aVF)

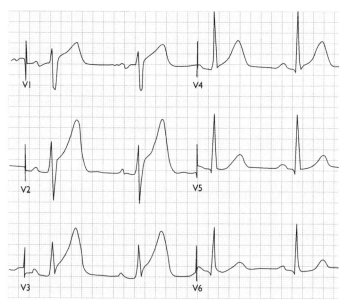

Figure 2.11: Anterior MI – ST elevation is seen in the anterior chest leads (V1–V4)

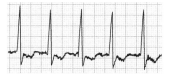

Figure 2.12: Supraventricular tachycardia (SVT) – note the absence of the P wave and the narrow QRS complex. The rate is between 150 and 200 bpm

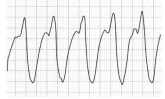

Figure 2.14: Broad complex tachycardia – ventricular tachycardia (VT). Note the rate (>100) and the broadness of the QRS complex

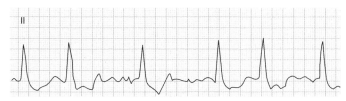

Figure 2.13: Fast atrial fibrillation (rate over 100). Note the irregular baseline and rate

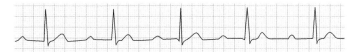

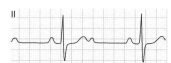

Figure 2.15: 1st degree heart block – prolonged PR interval

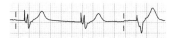

Figure 2.16: 2nd degree heart block – note the two P waves to every QRS complex

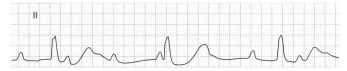

Figure 2.18: Paced complete heart block – note the small vertical lines before each QRS complex. When a patient is reliant on pacing it is very difficult to correctly interpret ECGs, e.g. if you are looking for ST changes

Figure 2.17: Complete (3rd degree) heart block – complete dissociation between the P waves and QRS complexes

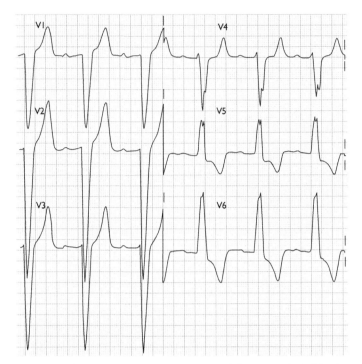

Figure 2.19: Left bundle branch block – note the 'W'-shaped QRS complexes in leads V1/2 and the 'M' shaped complex in V5/6

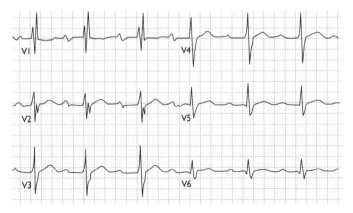

Figure 2.20: Trifascicular block – this is a combination of left axis deviation (LAD), right bundle branch block (RBBB) and 1st degree heart block (a P–R interval of >5s)

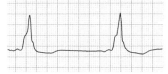

Figure 2.21: Wolff-Parkinson-White (WPW) syndrome – caused by an accessory pathway between the atria and the ventricles. There is a decreased P–R interval and a wide QRS complex. Note the slurred upstroke to the QRS complex (δ-wave) in the chest leads

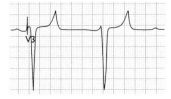

Figure 2.22: Hyperkalaemia – note the flattening of P waves, broad QRS complexes and tall, 'tented' T waves. This patient had potassium of 9 mmol/L

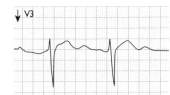

Figure 2.23: U wave – commonly seen in hypokalaemia. Note the small T waves

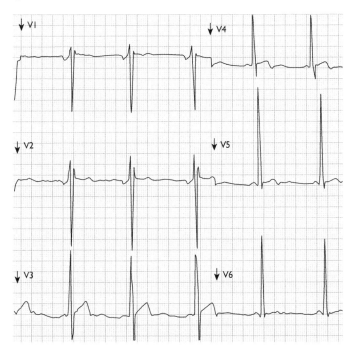

Figure 2.24: Left ventricular hypertrophy (LVH) – note the size of the S waves in V1 and the R wave in V6 (fulfils voltage criteria)

CARDIOVASCULAR

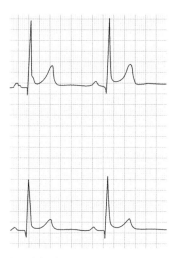

Figure 2.25: Pericarditis – note the global, 'saddle-shaped' ST elevation

Exercise tolerance test (ETT)

Exercise stress testing is both a diagnostic and a prognostic tool for assessing patients with suspected (e.g. symptoms of chest pain on exertion) or known (recent MI) ischaemic heart disease. As coronary blood flow increases during exercise to meet the higher myocardial metabolic demands, obstruction to the coronary blood flow results in ECG changes.

Indications
■ Assessment for signs of obstructive coronary artery disease in patients with chest pain.
■ Assessment of other symptoms (exertional presyncope) or signs (exertional arrhythmias).

■ Determine prognosis and management in symptomatic patients and those with a prior history of coronary heart disease (including those with medically/stent treated angina or post MI).
■ CHD screening in asymptomatic selected high-risk populations.

Commonly used protocol
■ Bruce protocol (or 'Modified' Bruce: post-acute coronary syndrome (ACS) / 'sedentary' patients).
■ Low risk (no ischaemia for 8–12 h), intermediate risk (no ischaemia for 2–3/7).
■ Four stages × 3 mins: increased workload by raising speed and incline of the treadmill.
■ Constant ECG record and blood pressure measured manually at each stage.
■ Protocol continued until one of several endpoints reached.
■ Maximum heart rate: 220 – age or 208 – (0.7 × age) (more reliable in older patients): 85% of maximum predicted heart rate = satisfactory.
NB: Drugs should be stopped before the test as these can give affect the outcome, e.g. beta blockers reduce the sensitivity of the test and digoxin gives an abnormal resting ECG with down-sloping ST changes in the lateral leads.

Report
■ HR/BP (max/min) response, ECG changes, symptoms reported, number of METs (metabolic equivalents) & functional class achieved, ectopics during or after exercise, maximum predicted HR achieved (should ideally be 85% or above)

■ 1 MET = amount of O_2 consumed at rest (3.5 mL O_2/kg/min). Average activity of daily living = 5 METs.

Normal ECG changes

■ P-wave height increase.
■ R- and T-wave height decrease.
■ J-point depression.
■ ST segment sharp upslope.
■ Q-T interval shortening.

Abnormal ECG changes

■ ST-segment depression (horizontal or downsloping) >1 mm (*NB:* Using 0.5 mm depression raises sensitivity and decreases specificity, with the opposite occurring if 2 mm depression used).

High probability of coronary artery disease

■ Horizontal ST depression ≥2 mm or downsloping ST depression or ST depression in ≥5 leads.
■ Early positive response within 5 minutes or persistent ST depression for ≥6 minutes into recovery.
■ Exertional hypotension.

Endpoints

■ Absolute: BP fall >20 mmHg systolic/ischaemia/pain/cyanosis/VT/patient request.
■ Relative: shortness of breath (SOB)/fatigue/HT (hypertensive) response/other arrhythmias.

Contraindications

■ Acute MI within past 4–6 days or unstable angina (rest pain) in past 48 h.
■ Uncontrolled hypertension (systolic BP >220 mmHg, diastolic BP >120 mmHg).
■ Severe aortic stenosis.

■ Severe hypertrophic obstructive cardiomyopathy.
■ Untreated life-threatening arrhythmia.
■ Dissecting aneurysm or very recent aortic surgery.
■ Uncontrolled heart failure.
■ Myocarditis/pericarditis.
■ Acute systemic infection.
■ Deep vein thrombosis (DVT).

Patients who are unsuitable for treadmill exercise test (e.g. reduced mobility, poor exercise capacity, atrial fibrillation or resting LBBB) can have other forms of non-invasive assessment of cardiac ischaemia. This usually takes the form of one of the following.

■ Dobutamine stress echocardiogram.
■ Adenosine or dobutamine myocardial perfusion imaging using radioactive isotopes such as thallium.

Cardiopulmonary exercise testing (CPET)

■ Cardiopulmonary exercise testing is an increasingly used, non-invasive and objective method of evaluating both cardiac and pulmonary function.
■ During exercise, a mouthpiece (pressure differential pneumotachygraph) samples the inspired and expired gas, allowing both the oxygen uptake and carbon dioxide elimination to be computed.
■ ECG treadmill studies focus on detection of ischaemia, whereas CPET allows measurement of ventricular, respiratory and cellular function via the measurement of gas exchange.
■ CPET can be used to evaluate cardiac function (e.g. during the investigation and management of cardiac disease). Respiratory function may be evaluated dynamically by exercise

spirometry thus detecting exercise-induced asthma as well as restrictive and obstructive lung disease.

Tilt-table testing

■ This test is useful in the investigation of symptoms such as dizziness and syncope.

■ Patients are strapped on to a table that can be rotated so that they can be positioned anywhere from standing upright to lying with their head tilted backwards and downwards.

■ By tilting the patient's body to a variety of angles, the patient's symptoms can be recorded, as can readings of BP and ECG.

■ While a healthy individual can compensate for changes in posture, those with impaired autonomic function can experience postural (orthostatic) hypotension.

■ Although this is usually a safe procedure (aside from the induction of symptoms such as dizziness/syncope), on rare occasions tilt-table testing can induce asystole or seizures.

■ Orthostatic hypotension can be due to a number of factors, including:

• hypovolaemia (e.g. dehydration)

• age-related (increasing incidence with increasing age)

• autonomic dysfunction (e.g. related to complications of diabetes mellitus or multisystem atrophy (Shy-Drager syndrome))

• cardiac causes (e.g. arrhythmias or structural disorders)

• secondary to drugs (e.g. antihypertensives).

■ There are two predominant types of positive responses during tilt-table testing.

• Cardioinhibitory response: development of significant bradycardia or asystole with subsequent hypotension. These patients may benefit from permanent pacemaker implantation to prevent symptoms/syncope.

• Vasodepressor response: development of significant hypotension with relative preservation of heart rate leading to symptoms/syncope. These patients are unlikely to benefit from permanent pacing.

• There can also be a mixed picture of the above two responses.

Lying and standing blood pressures

■ In a more routine clinical setting, it is common practice for lying and standing blood pressure measurements to be taken.

■ In healthy patients there is normally little difference between lying and standing blood pressures.

■ However, a significant fall (20 mmHg or more) can occur in older people, patients with diabetes and those with symptoms suggestive of postural hypotension.

Cardiac enzymes

Cardiac enzymes are a group of blood-based markers that can be used to help determine if cardiac damage has taken place. They should always be used in conjunction with the clinical history, examination and other relevant investigations. A few such markers are discussed below.

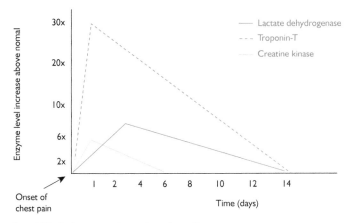

Figure 2.26: Cardiac enzyme changes observed post-MI

Creatine kinase (CK)

This enzyme is found in muscle. Several iso-forms exist: heart muscle (CK-MB), skeletal muscle (CK-MM) and brain (CK-BB). CK is raised in over 90% of myocardial infarctions. It:

■ rises 3–6 h after injury
■ peaks at 18 h
■ returns to baseline at 48/72 h.

It is particularly of use in patients with conditions that could cause false positive troponin elevations (e.g. pulmonary embolus, renal failure). In these patients, it can be useful to use a combination of troponin and CK together.

Other causes of a raised CK
■ Rhabdomyolysis (including with physical exertion and muscle trauma)
■ Defibrillation
■ Polymyositis/Dermatomyositis
■ Surgery
■ Muscular dystrophy

■ Bowel ischaemia
■ Statin therapy
■ Convulsions

Lactate dehydrogenase (LDH)

These days, this enzyme is rarely measured post-MI. It:

■ rises 10 h after injury
■ peaks at 24–48 h
■ returns to baseline after 12–14 days.

Other causes of a raised LDH
■ Haemolysis
■ Hepatocyte damage
■ Pulmonary embolus
■ Tumour necrosis

Myoglobin

An enzyme found in striated muscle and released by damage to skeletal or cardiac muscle. It:

■ rises early (1–4 h post-injury)

- peaks at 6–8 h
- returns to baseline after around 24 h.

Aspartate transaminase (AST)

Similar to alanine transaminase, the GOT1 isoenzyme of AST is found in cardiac muscle cells and is released upon damage of the tissue. It:

- rises 18–24 h after injury
- peaks at 48 h
- returns to baseline at 72 h.

Other causes of a raised AST

- Liver disease
- Skeletal muscle damage
- Haemolysis

Troponin I and T

These are the contractile proteins of the myofibril and the preferred markers for clinical use. Presence of these cardiac iso-forms is very sensitive and specific for cardiac injury. The 'T' form is probably more commonly used by most laboratories. It:

- rises after 3–8 h
- peaks at 12–18 h
- remains elevated for 7–10 days.

Other causes of a raised troponin (>0.01)

- Renal failure
- Pulmonary embolus
- Stroke
- Sepsis

Infective endocarditis

Endocarditis should be considered whenever there is fever associated with a new onset murmur. Half of all cases occur in normal valves, with the cases on abnormal valves (valvular disease/ prosthetic valves, etc.) running a subacute course.

Organisms responsible

Any cause of bacteraemia (e.g. dental or invasive urinary procedure). Causes include the following.

- *Streptococcus viridans* (commonest)
- *Enterococcus*
- *Staphylococcus aureus/epidermidis*
- Microaerophillic *streptococcus*
- Diphtherioids
- HACEK Gram negative organisms (*Haemophillus, Actinobacillus, Cardiobacterium, Eikenella, Kingella*)

Non-bacterial causes

- Systemic lupus erythematosus (SLE, Libman-Sacks endocarditis)
- Malignancy

Diagnosis

Essential investigations include the following.

- Blood cultures: at least three sets of blood cultures taken at different times and from different sites.
- Transthoracic echocardiography (TTE): required to identify the valvular vegetations that characterise endocarditis (although this cannot be excluded on TTE and transoesophageal echo (TOE) is frequently required for the diagnosis).

Dukes' criteria

Two major, or one major and three minor, or five minor criteria.

Major criteria

- Positive blood culture (typical organism in two different culture bottles, or persistently positive cultures).
- Evidence for endocardial involvement (vegetation/dehiscence of prosthetic valve, abscess on echo) or new valvular regurgitation (echo, not clinical assessment).

Minor criteria

- Predisposing heart condition/intravenous drug abuse.
- Fever: temperature >38°C.
- Vascular phenomena: septic emboli, arterial embolic disease, infarctions, others.
- Immunologic phenomena: glomerulonephritis, rheumatoid factor, others.
- Microbiological evidence (cultures not meeting major criteria).
- Echo evidence (not meeting major criteria).

Rheumatic fever

This is a systemic infection that can occur a few weeks after pharyngeal infection with Group A beta-haemolytic *streptococcus*. The cause is antigenic mimicry (antibody to bacterial cell wall cross-reacting to heart valve tissue). In developed countries, the incidence is about 2–14 cases per 100,000, so it is a rare disease.

Modified Jones criteria

Evidence of recent streptococcal infection and two major, or one major and two minor criteria.

Evidence of recent infection

- Positive throat swab.

- Raised ASOT (anti-streptolysin O titre) >200 u/mL or DNAase B-titre.
- History of scarlet fever.

Major

- **J**oints (migratory polyarthritis): temporary migrating inflammation of large joints (usually starts in the legs and migrates upwards).
- **O**bvious (carditis): inflammation of the cardiac muscle – manifests as congestive heart failure (shortness of breath), pericarditis (rub), new heart murmur, tachycardia or conduction abnormalities.
- **N**odules (subcutaneous nodules, a type of Aschoff body): painless collections of firm, mobile collagen fibres on the backs of the wrist/outside of the elbow/front of the knees.
- **E**rythema marginatum: rash that begins on the arms/trunk and spreads outward to form a raised ring with a central clearing. Almost never starts on the face and worsens with heat.
- **S**ydenham's chorea (St Vitus' dance): characteristic series of rapid, non-purposeful movements of the arms and head (can occur very late in the disease process). Can be associated with uncharacteristic behaviour.

Minor

- Fever.
- Arthralgia (joint pain without swelling).
- Laboratory test abnormalities: raised ESR/CRP/leucocytosis.
- ECG abnormalities: prolonged PR interval.
- Evidence of Group A Streptococcal infection: positive cultures/elevated or rising ASOT.
- Previous rheumatic fever or inactive heart disease.

Valves affected

Complications can affect:

■ mitral (70%)
■ aortic (40%)
■ tricuspid (10%)
■ pulmonary (2%).

Pressures and sounds

Arterial blood pressure (ABP)

■ This is the force exerted on the arterial walls by circulating blood.

■ It has two components: 'systolic' (peak arterial pressure) and 'diastolic' (lowest arterial pressure). The average pressure throughout the cardiac cycle is the 'mean arterial pressure'.

■ ABP is commonly measured using a sphygmomanometer. This involves inflation of a cuff around the upper arm to occlude flow. The examiner then releases pressure in the cuff while auscultating over the brachial artery for Korotkoff sounds (produced by turbulent flow as blood flow returns). The pressure reading when the first Korotkoff sound is heard is the systolic pressure. The cuff pressure is then further released until no sound is heard (fifth Korotkoff sound) – this is diastolic pressure.

■ Ambulatory BP monitoring involves the use of an automated sphygmomanometer to monitor ABP over a fixed period, e.g. 24 h. This can provide a representation of BP variation over time in a more realistic environment for a patient.

■ Arterial line placement (cannulation of an artery, e.g. radial) is an invasive technique for more accurately measuring ABP. This method also allows the

beat-by-beat pressure waveform to be visualised.

> *Normal ranges (these vary between healthy adults):* Systolic = 110–130 mmHg, Diastolic = 70–90 mmHg

24-hour (ambulatory) BP

■ This involves the use of a cuff that takes BP readings at set intervals (e.g. every 20 minutes during the day and less frequently at night).

■ It can be useful in certain patients (e.g. those with borderline readings, poorly controlled/labile hypertension, suspected white-coat (or reverse white-coat) hypertension, etc.)

■ Ambulatory BP recording is not commonly used, as there is still a limited evidence-base for its applicability. There is some evidence to suggest that higher ambulatory BP readings are associated with a higher risk of mortality.

■ Average ambulatory values recorded can commonly be lower than clinic recordings, as the effect of 'white coat hypertension' can be reduced by recording BP in a more natural environment for the patient. Conversely, some patients may have a reverse white-coat effect (with higher values during the day than are noted in individual clinic readings).

Mean arterial pressure (MAP)

■ This is the average arterial blood pressure over a cardiac cycle – effectively the perfusion pressure of target organs (i.e. the area under a pressure-time curve).

- In practice, MAP can be estimated using the following:
- MAP = cardiac output × systemic vascular resistance
- MAP = (2/3 × diastolic pressure) + (1/3 × systolic pressure), which can also be expressed as: diastolic pressure + (1/3 × (systolic − diastolic pressure)).

NB: Remember: Cardiac output = heart rate × stroke volume.

Intra-cardiac pressures and O_2 saturations

Site	Pressure (mmHg)	O_2 saturation
Inferior vena cava	(approximately similar to right atrium)	76%
Superior vena cava	(approximately similar to right atrium)	70%
Right atrium	0–8	74%
Right ventricle	15–30 (sys), 0–8 (end dias)	74%
Pulmonary artery	15–30 (sys), 5–15 (dias), mean (10–20), wedge (3–15)	74%
Left ventricle	80–140 (sys), 60–90 (end dias)	98%
Aorta	80–140 (sys), 60–90 (dias), 70–100 (mean)	98%

(Adapted from the Oxford Handbook of Clinical Medicine, Cardiology section)

JVP components
- a = atrial contraction (right atrium systole)
- c = tricuspid valve closure
- x-descent = ventricular systole (fall in atrial pressure), atrial diastole
- v = atrial filling (closed tricuspid valve)
- y-descent = tricuspid valve opening

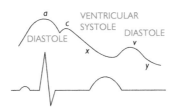

Figure 2.27: Components of the jugular venous pressure (JVP)

Timings and pressures

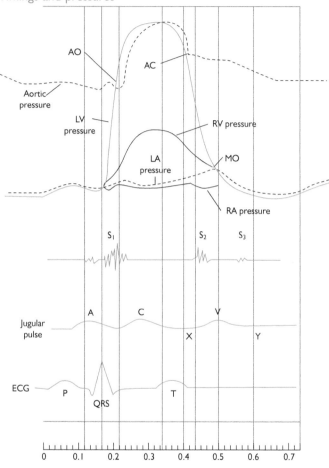

Figure 2.28: Relationship between the cardiac pressures and the ECG

AO = aortic valve opening

Anachrotic notch: presystolic rise prior to aortic valve opening, during isovolumetric contraction

AC: aortic valve closure

MO: mitral valve opening

Ventricular systole

■ Isovolumetric contraction (after closure of the mitral valve and before opening of the aortic valve) = rapid rise in pressure until it exceeds that of aortic pressure and aortic valve opens.

■ Ejection phase (opening to the closing of the aortic valve) = blood flows into aorta until aortic valve closure.

Ventricular diastole

■ Relaxation of ventricle (aortic valve closes and mitral valve opens, allowing ventricular filling).

■ Diastasis: later, slower period of filling when left ventricle is nearly full. Pressure in left ventricle = pressure in left atrium (filling continues until ejection occurs).

Central venous pressure (CVP)

■ In the clinical setting, CVP, measured using a venous catheter, can be used as an indicator of cardiac output.

■ Cardiac output is a function of venous return, heart rate, cardiac contractility and peripheral vascular resistance.

■ Although CVP does not solely reflect intravascular volume (hence isolated readings are not so useful, with a 'normal' resting CVP ranging from 0 to 10 mmHg), changes in CVP can be used to guide treatment.

■ For example, CVP can rise with pathologies (e.g. heart failure, tension pneumothorax, pulmonary embolism).

■ As an approximate reflection of right ventricular end-diastolic volume (right ventricular preload), CVP measurements can be used to guide intravenous fluid replacement.

■ In practice, the CVP response can be used to evaluate the response to a fluid bolus (e.g. 200–250 mL); this should result in a transient, small rise in CVP in the hypovolaemic patient (whereas the same bolus will result in a larger response in the normovolaemic patient).

Other cardiac investigations

Echocardiography

(See Chapter 15)

Cardiac magnetic resonance imaging (MRI)

Cardiac MRI is an increasingly popular non-invasive procedure. It allows visualisation and measurement of the structure of the cardiac chambers. It can also provide a non-invasive method of visualising the coronary vessels and assessing the extent of thrombosis.

Although cardiac MRI has a lower spatial resolution than computed tomography (CT), it has superior temporal and contrast resolution. Applications include the investigation of structural conditions (e.g. congenital heart disease) and cardiomyopathy (e.g. hypertrophic cardiomyopathy), as well as coronary artery imaging and assessment of myocardial perfusion.

Cardiac catheterisation

This procedure allows direct visualisation of the coronary vessels.

■ The right heart is usually cannulated through the femoral vein and the catheter is passed to the heart using a guide wire. The left heart can be cannulated through the femoral artery.

■ Access to the left heart and coronary arteries is usually gained via the femoral artery using specially designed catheters, which are passed over guidewires. Right heart studies are performed via the femoral vein.

■ Access via the radial or brachial artery has recently become more fashionable among cardiologists because of fewer bleeding complications and earlier patient ambulation.

■ Characteristic pressure waveforms can indicate the site of the tip of the catheter. Abnormal pressures can help diagnose certain pathologies (e.g. valvular disease).

■ Measurements that can be made include: pressures (right/left chambers, pulmonary vessels, pulmonary capillary wedge pressures, etc.), oxygen partial pressures (concentration), cardiac output (using Fick principle).

■ Angiography is undertaken by the use of a contrast medium and radiological imaging.

■ Coronary artery stenting is the main therapeutic application, and recently percutaneous aortic valve implantation has become a realistic option in the treatment of aortic stenosis (although this method is still in its infancy).

■ Complications include vessel damage, thrombo-embolus formation, arrhythmia and haemorrhage.

■ There is increasing interest in assessment of coronary arteries using CT angiography, which, using 64-slice and more recently 256-slice technology allows excellent spatial resolution of the coronary arteries.

Cardiac electrophysiology

This specialist procedure can be used in the investigation and treatment of conduction defects, especially those that are refractory to drug therapy, e.g. paroxysmal atrial fibrillation. It involves the use of catheters to record electrical activity within the heart. This technique can help detect abnormal conduction pathways, which can also be ablated ('burnt away' using radiofrequency energy ablation) to terminate their activity. Examples include accessory pathway mapping and ablation in patients with the Wolff-Parkinson-White syndrome.

Peripheral vascular disease

When investigating peripheral arterial disease, aside from detailed clinical history and examination, a number of other general investigations can be of use. These include the following.

Blood

While none of these blood investigations are diagnostic, they can be helpful as part of an overall assessment.

■ Full blood count (?anaemia, ?polycythaemia)

■ Urea and electrolytes (?renal disease)

■ CRP/ESR (?vasculitis, ?inflammatory aortic aneurysm)

■ Cholesterol and lipid profile (general cardiovascular disease risk factors)

■ Auto-antibodies (?vasculitis).

Other

■ Urinalysis (?glucose, ?diabetes mellitus)

■ Chest x-ray (?cardiac pathology, e.g. dilated atria as source of emboli)

■ ECG (?cardiac pathology, ?arrhythmia – could send off emboli)

■ Cardiac echocardiogram (either transthoracic or transoesophageal – ?embolic source such as abnormal valve)

■ Ankle brachial pressure index *(see below)*

■ Abdominal and carotid/peripheral vascular Doppler ultrasound/contrast angiography (see *Chapter 15 for more details*)

Ankle Brachial Pressure Index (ABPI)

■ An ABPI is a quick, simple, non-invasive method of measuring the effect that arterial disease is having on the blood pressure in the lower leg.

■ If there is arterial disease in the arteries of the leg the blood pressure at the foot is reduced. The degree of reduction of the blood pressure is a measure of the severity of the arterial disease.

Method

■ A doppler probe is used to locate the ankle peripheral pulse (using a foot vessel, e.g. posterior tibial or dorsalis pedis).

■ A sphygmomanometer is inflated over the calf (proximal to the probe) until the pulse is occluded.

■ The cuff is slowly deflated and the pressure at the instant the pulse returns is recorded. This is the systolic blood pressure reading for that vessel. The higher pressure between the left and right legs is recorded.

■ The procedure is repeated with the brachial artery (arm) to obtain the systolic blood pressure.

Normal ranges
(These are a guide only)

>1.2	Abnormal vessel hardening (e.g. diabetes, peripheral vascular disease)
0.9–1.2	Normal range
0.8–0.9	Mild arterial disease
0.5–0.9	Moderate arterial disease (likely to have signs/symptoms of intermittent claudication)
<0.5	Severe arterial disease (may have signs/symptoms of critical ischaemia)

Chapter 3
RESPIRATORY

Introduction

A range of symptoms, from shortness of breath to cough, may warrant further investigation of the respiratory tract. As for a number of other specialties discussed in this book, imaging – for example in the form of a chest x-ray or CT scan – plays an important role in assessment. Beyond this, there are a number of unique investigative modalities that can be employed. In this chapter, we will consider some of the tools more commonly used in clinical practice.

Topics covered
- Asthma
- Peak expiratory flow rate
- Spirometry
- Lung volumes
- Flow-volume loops
- Acid-base balance
- Anion gap
- Arterial blood gas (ABG)

- Respiratory failure
- Alveolar-arterial (A-a) gradient calculation
- Pneumonia severity
- Pulmonary embolism
- Pleural effusion
- Pulmonary fibrosis
- Tumours of the lung
- Other tests

Asthma

Definition and background

- Asthma is a chronic condition involving reversible airways obstruction.
- Airway inflammation and other features, such as mucus plugging, can be in response to a number of triggers. These can range from environmental stimuli (allergens, cold weather, etc.) to exertion.

- Categorising the severity of both, acute and chronic asthma is important in determining optimal management.
- The table below provides an example of how to objectively determine severity. Note that the values provided should only be used as a guide – they are not universally agreed as definitive criteria.

The hands-on guide to data interpretation. By S. Abraham, K. Kulkarni, R. Madhu and D. Provan. Published 2010 by Blackwell Publishing Ltd.

Determining severity (acute attack)

Features	Mild	Moderate	Severe	Life-threatening
O₂ saturations (initial)	>95%	92–95%	<92%	<92%
PEFR/FEV1 (% of predicted/ best)	>75%	>50–75%	33–50%	<33%
pH	Respiratory alkalosis (>7.45)	Respiratory alkalosis (>7.45)	Normalising	Respiratory acidosis (<7.35)
PaO₂	Normal	Normal	Decreasing	Low –<8 kPa (<60 mmHg)
PaCO₂	Low (<4.6 kPa; <35 mmHg)	Low (< 4.6 kPa; <35 mmHg)	Rising	Normal – raised (4.6–6 kPa; 35–45 mmHg)
Pulse rate	<100/min	100–110/min	≥110/min	≥110/min
Pulsus paradoxus	<10 mmHg (not palpable)	10–20 mmHg (may be palpable)	20–40 mmHg (palpable)	
Respiratory rate (resp/min)	<20	>20	≥25	Decreasing
Speech	Normal sentences	Uses shorter sentences	Unable to complete sentences in one breath	Quiet and tired
Mental state (orientation)	Alert	Alert but irritable	Increasing irritability, decreasing alertness	Confusion/coma
Cyanosis	None	Possible cyanosis	Likely cyanosis	Cyanosis
Strength of breathing	Normal	Normal (increased intercostal retractions/ accessory muscle use)	Tiring (increased intercostal retractions/ accessory muscle use)	Exhausted (feeble respiratory effort), silent chest, wheeze less audible

1 mmHg = 037.133 kPa
(Table adapted from the British Thoracic Society's 2008 Guidelines)

Other categories:
■ **Near-fatal asthma:** raised PaCO₂ and/or requiring mechanical ventilation with raised inflation pressures.
■ **Brittle asthma:**
• Type 1: wide PEF variability (>40% diurnal variation for >50% of the time over a period >150 days) despite intense therapy.
• Type 2: sudden severe attacks on a background of apparently well controlled asthma.

Determining severity (chronic asthma)

Note that the stratification below is not as commonly used in clinical practice as the tables above (for acute asthma). However, the categories do provide a broad indication of how to classify the severity of chronic asthma to help determine appropriate management.

Feature	Mild	Moderate	Severe
Symptoms (wheeze, chest tightness, cough, dyspnoea)	Occasionally (e.g. post-infection/ exercise)	Most days	Every day
Nocturnal symptoms	No	<1x/week	>1x/ week
Frequency of symptoms	<2x/wk	Daily	Continual
Early morning symptoms	No	<1x/week	>1x/ week
Emergency visit to hospital due to symptoms?	No	Occasionally	Often
Previous 'life-threatening' attack (required ICU admission or ventilation)	No	Usually not	Likely history
Bronchodilator use	<2x/week	Most days	>3–4x/ day
FEV₁/PEFR (% predicted)	>80%	60–80%	<60%
Current morning PEFR (upon waking)	>90% best	80–90% best	<80% best
PEFR variability	<20–30%	>30%	>30%
Activity limitation	None/minimal	Noticeable impact	Severely limited

PEFR = peak expiratory flow rate, FEV1 = forced expiratory volume (in 1 second). See later in the chapter for more detailed explanation of these terms.

Peak expiratory flow rate (PEFR)

Definition

This is a simple investigation for estimating the degree of airway obstruction, commonly used in monitoring patients with asthma over both the long and short term.

How is it measured?

■ The marker on the peak-flow meter should be reset to 0, and a clean mouthpiece attached.

PEFR is then measured by asking patients to first 'breathe all the way out', then 'breathe all the way in', then place their mouth in a tight seal around the inlet of a peak-flow meter and 'blow out as hard as they can'. This should be done while standing.

The best of three readings should be used.

Peak-flow meters are cheap and simple to use. PEFR readings are particularly useful when trends are compared; asking patients to keep a diary of PEFR readings over a period of time is therefore important.

Predicted PEFR measurements

PEFR can very with age, sex, height and ethnicity.

Note: Height in the graph below is in cm.

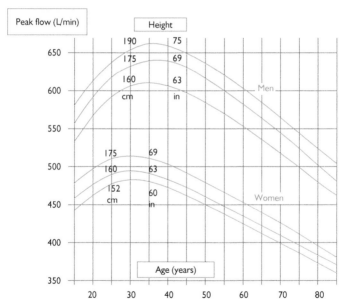

Figure 3.1: Predicted PEFR

PEFR measurement tables

PEFR can vary with age, sex and height. The example table below shows the variation in PEFR based on these criteria.

Height (cm)

Age (years)	Males											Females										
	145	150	155	160	165	170	175	180	185	190	195	130	135	140	145	150	155	160	165	170	175	180
Wright scale (L/min)																						
15	492	508	524	541	557	573	589	605	621	637	653	362	376	390	404	418	432	446	460	474	488	502
20	514	530	546	562	578	595	611	627	643	659	675	370	384	398	412	426	440	454	468	482	496	510
25	528	545	561	577	593	609	625	641	657	673	689	378	392	406	420	434	447	461	475	489	503	517
30	537	553	569	585	601	617	633	649	665	681	698	384	397	411	425	439	453	467	481	495	509	523
35	539	555	571	587	603	619	636	652	668	684	700	387	401	415	429	443	457	471	485	499	513	527
40	537	553	569	585	601	617	633	649	665	682	698	389	403	417	431	445	459	473	487	501	515	528
45	530	546	563	579	595	611	627	643	659	675	691	388	402	416	430	444	458	471	485	499	513	527
50	521	537	553	569	585	601	618	634	650	666	682	383	397	411	425	439	453	467	481	495	509	523
55	509	525	541	557	574	590	606	622	638	654	670	375	389	403	417	431	445	459	473	487	501	515
60	496	512	528	544	560	577	593	609	625	641	657	363	377	391	405	419	433	446	460	474	488	502
65	482	498	514	530	547	563	579	595	611	627	643	346	360	374	388	402	416	430	443	457	471	485
70	469	485	501	517	533	549	565	581	597	613	630	324	338	352	366	380	394	407	421	435	449	463
75	456	472	488	504	520	536	552	569	585	601	617	296	310	324	338	352	366	380	394	408	422	436
80	445	461	477	493	509	526	542	558	574	590	606	263	277	291	305	318	332	346	360	374	388	402
85	437	453	469	485	501	517	533	550	566	582	598	223	237	251	265	279	292	306	320	334	348	362

Height (cm)

Age (years)	Males											Females										
	145	150	155	160	165	170	175	180	185	190	195	130	135	140	145	150	155	160	165	170	175	180
American Thoracic Society Scale (L/min)																						
15	447	470	493	515	538	561	583	606	629	651	674	296	313	329	345	361	378	394	410	426	443	459
20	480	502	525	548	571	593	616	639	661	684	707	307	323	340	356	372	388	405	421	437	453	470
25	501	524	546	569	592	615	637	660	683	705	728	316	332	348	365	381	397	413	430	446	462	478
30	513	535	556	581	603	626	649	671	694	717	740	323	339	355	371	388	404	420	436	453	469	485
35	516	538	561	584	606	629	652	674	697	720	743	327	343	360	376	392	408	425	441	457	473	490
40	512	534	557	580	602	625	648	671	693	716	739	328	345	361	377	393	410	426	442	458	475	491
45	502	525	548	570	593	616	638	661	684	707	729	327	343	359	375	392	408	424	440	457	473	489
50	489	511	534	557	579	602	625	648	670	693	716	321	338	354	370	386	403	419	435	451	468	484
55	472	495	518	540	563	586	608	631	654	677	699	312	328	345	361	377	393	410	426	442	458	475
60	455	477	500	523	545	568	591	614	636	659	682	299	315	331	347	364	380	396	412	429	445	461
65	437	460	482	505	528	551	573	596	619	641	664	280	297	313	329	345	362	378	394	410	427	443
70	421	444	466	489	512	535	557	580	603	625	648	257	274	290	306	322	339	355	371	387	404	420
75	408	431	453	476	499	521	544	567	590	612	635	229	245	261	278	294	310	326	343	359	375	391
80	199	422	445	467	490	513	535	558	581	604	626	195	211	227	243	260	276	292	308	325	341	357
85	396	419	442	464	487	510	532	555	578	601	623	155	171	181	203	220	236	252	268	285	301	317

RESPIRATORY

Diurnal variation

■ PEFR in normal subjects can exhibit the phenomenon of 'diurnal variation', with lower PEFRs in the mornings and higher rates during the evenings.

■ This variation can be exaggerated in patients with asthma, with consistent variations of >20% being suggestive of a diagnosis of asthma. This number can rise during acute exacerbations.

■ The diurnal variability should be considered in the overall management, with patients taking their own 'diary' measurements at these times in order that this variation is recorded.

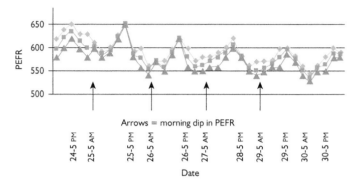

Figure 3.2: Diurnal variation in PEFR

Spirometry

■ This technique allows a far more detailed assessment of respiratory function to be made.

■ Also commonly referred to as lung or pulmonary function tests, spirometry records the volume and flow rate of inhaled and exhaled air to determine several measures of lung function.

■ Chronic obstructive pulmonary disease (COPD) and pulmonary fibrosis are two conditions that are commonly investigated using spirometry.

■ By producing volume-time and flow-volume loops, a key use of spirometry is to distinguish between obstructive and restrictive lung defects.

Obstructive versus restrictive defects

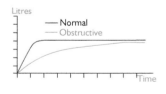

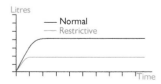

Figure 3.3: Appearance of obstructive and restrictive defects on spirometry

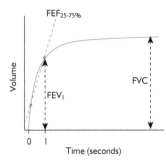

Figure 3.4: Measures used in spirometry

Measure	Full name	Definition
FVC	Forced vital capacity	The maximum volume of air that can be expired in a single complete expiration
FEV_1	Forced expiratory volume in 1 sec	Maximum volume of air that can be expired in 1 sec
FEV_1/FVC	Ratio of FEV_1:FVC	Used to determine if airway abnormality is restrictive or obstructive
K_{CO}	Carbon monoxide gas transfer coefficient	Diffusion of CO from the alveoli into the pulmonary capillary blood (not measured by spirometry – requires lung function laboratory) Low = emphysema, interstitial lung disease, pulmonary oedema or embolus, anaemia High = pulmonary haemorrhage, polycythaemia

- Normal FEV_1/FVC ratio ≈75–80%
- Obstructive
- FEV_1/FVC ratio <75% (FEV_1 reduced more than FVC)
- hyperinflation (increased total lung capacity, TLC, and residual volume, RV)
- e.g. asthma, COPD
- Restrictive
- FEV_1/FVC ratio normal/slightly raised (FVC reduced more than FEV_1)
- reduced lung volumes (decreased TLC and RV)
- e.g. pulmonary fibrosis, sarcoidosis, kyphoscoliosis (neuromuscular problems).

Predicted FEV_1/FVC volumes

The following tables provide data on predicted FEV_1 and FVC volumes. Note that these 'normal values' are dependent on age, sex and race.

FEV$_1$ (litres)						Male					
Height (cm)	145	150	155	160	165	170	175	180	185	190	195
Age 10	2.31	2.54	2.77	3.00	3.23	3.46	3.69	3.92	4.15	4.38	4.61
12	2.40	2.63	2.86	3.09	3.32	3.55	3.78	4.01	4.24	4.47	4.70
14	2.49	2.72	2.95	3.18	3.41	3.64	3.87	4.10	4.33	4.56	4.79
16	2.58	2.81	3.04	3.27	3.50	3.73	3.96	4.19	4.42	4.65	4.88
18	2.67	2.90	3.13	3.36	3.59	3.82	4.05	4.28	4.51	4.74	4.97
20	2.76	2.99	3.22	3.45	3.68	3.91	4.14	4.37	4.60	4.83	5.06
25	2.66	2.92	3.18	3.44	3.70	3.96	4.22	4.48	4.74	5.00	5.26
30	2.53	2.79	3.05	3.31	3.57	3.83	4.09	4.35	4.61	4.87	5.13
40	2.26	2.52	2.78	3.04	3.30	3.56	3.82	4.08	4.34	4.60	4.86
50	1.99	2.25	2.51	2.77	3.03	3.29	3.55	3.81	4.07	4.33	4.59
60	1.72	1.98	2.24	2.50	2.76	3.02	3.28	3.54	3.80	4.06	4.32
70	1.45	1.71	1.97	2.23	2.49	2.75	3.01	3.27	3.53	3.79	4.05
80	1.18	1.44	1.70	1.96	2.22	2.48	2.74	3.00	3.26	3.52	3.78

FEV$_1$ (litres)

						Female					
Height (cm)	145	150	155	160	165	170	175	180	185	190	195
Age 10	2.06	2.20	2.33	2.47	2.60	2.74	2.87	3.01	3.14	3.28	3.41
12	2.23	2.37	2.50	2.64	2.77	2.91	3.04	3.18	3.31	3.45	3.58
14	2.40	2.54	2.67	2.81	2.94	3.08	3.21	3.35	3.48	3.62	3.75
16	2.57	2.71	2.84	2.98	3.11	3.25	3.38	3.52	3.65	3.79	3.92
18	2.74	2.88	3.01	3.15	3.28	3.42	3.55	3.69	3.82	3.96	4.09
20	2.70	2.84	2.97	3.11	3.24	3.38	3.51	3.65	3.78	3.92	4.05
25	2.60	2.73	2.87	3.00	3.14	3.27	3.41	3.54	3.68	3.81	3.95
30	2.49	2.63	2.76	2.90	3.03	3.17	3.30	3.44	3.57	3.71	3.84
40	2.28	2.42	2.55	2.69	2.82	2.96	3.09	3.23	3.36	3.50	3.63
50	2.07	2.21	2.34	2.48	2.61	2.75	2.88	3.02	3.15	3.29	3.42
60	1.86	2.00	2.13	2.27	2.40	2.54	2.67	2.81	2.94	3.08	3.21
70	1.65	1.79	1.92	2.06	2.19	2.33	2.46	2.60	2.73	2.87	3.00
80	1.44	1.58	1.71	1.85	1.98	2.12	2.25	2.39	2.52	2.66	2.79

Predicted FVC volumes

FVC (Litres)

Height (cm)						Male					
Age	145	150	155	160	165	170	175	180	185	190	195
10	2.52	2.77	3.02	3.27	3.52	3.77	4.02	4.27	4.52	4.77	5.02
12	2.68	2.93	3.18	3.43	3.68	3.93	4.18	4.43	4.68	4.93	5.18
14	2.83	3.08	3.33	3.58	3.83	4.08	4.33	4.58	4.83	5.08	5.33
16	2.99	3.24	3.49	3.74	3.99	4.24	4.49	4.74	4.99	5.24	5.49
18	3.15	3.40	3.65	3.90	4.15	4.40	4.65	4.90	5.15	5.40	5.65
20	3.30	3.55	3.80	4.05	4.30	4.55	4.80	5.05	5.30	5.55	5.80
25	3.24	3.57	3.89	4.22	4.54	4.87	5.19	5.52	5.84	6.17	6.49
30	3.10	3.42	3.75	4.07	4.40	4.72	5.05	5.37	5.70	6.02	6.35
40	2.81	3.13	3.46	3.78	4.11	4.43	4.76	5.08	5.41	5.73	6.06
50	2.52	2.84	3.17	3.49	3.82	4.14	4.47	4.79	5.12	5.44	5.77
60	2.23	2.55	2.88	3.20	3.53	3.85	4.18	4.50	4.83	5.15	5.48
70	1.94	2.26	2.59	2.91	3.24	3.56	3.89	4.21	4.54	4.86	5.19
80	1.65	1.97	2.30	2.62	2.95	3.27	3.60	3.92	4.25	4.57	4.90

FVC (litres)						Female					
Height (cm)	145	150	155	160	165	170	175	180	185	190	195
Age 10	2.24	2.40	2.57	2.73	2.90	3.06	3.23	3.39	3.56	3.72	3.89
12	2.42	2.59	2.75	2.92	3.08	3.25	3.41	3.58	3.74	3.91	4.07
14	2.60	2.77	2.93	3.10	3.26	3.43	3.59	3.76	3.92	4.09	4.25
16	2.79	2.95	3.12	3.28	3.45	3.61	3.78	3.94	4.11	4.27	4.44
18	2.97	3.14	3.30	3.47	3.63	3.80	3.96	4.13	4.29	4.46	4.62
20	3.15	3.34	3.52	3.71	3.89	4.08	4.26	4.45	4.63	4.82	5.00
25	3.04	3.23	3.41	3.60	3.78	3.97	4.15	4.34	4.52	4.71	4.89
30	2.93	3.12	3.30	3.49	3.67	3.86	4.04	4.23	4.41	4.60	4.78
40	2.71	2.90	3.08	3.27	3.45	3.64	3.82	4.01	4.19	4.38	4.56
50	2.49	2.68	2.86	3.05	3.23	3.42	3.60	3.79	3.97	4.16	4.34
60	2.27	2.46	2.64	2.83	3.01	3.20	3.38	3.57	3.75	3.94	4.12
70	2.05	2.24	2.42	2.61	2.79	2.98	3.16	3.35	3.53	3.72	3.90
80	1.83	2.02	2.20	2.39	2.57	2.76	2.94	3.13	3.31	3.50	3.68

(These four tables from www.nationalasthma.org.au/html/management/spiro_book/sp_bk010.asp#Mean)

Lung volumes

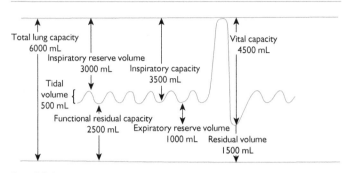

Figure 3.5: Lung volumes and capacities

A number of factors affect lung volumes, including sex, height, smoking status, physical fitness and altitude of residence. The values in the table below are for an average 70 kg male.

Measurement	Normal value	Calculation	Details
Total lung capacity (TLC)	6 L	IRV + TV + ERV + RV	Volume of gas in lung at end of maximal inspiration
Vital capacity (VC)	4.6 L	IRV + TV + ERV	Complete amount of air that can be forced out of lungs after end of maximal inspiration
Forced vital capacity (FVC)	4.8 L	(Spirometry)	Maximal amount of air that can be forced out of lungs after maximal inspiration
Tidal volume (TV)	500 mL	(Spirometry)	Volume of air breathed in and out during normal respiration
Residual volume (RV)	1.2 L	(Spirometry)	Volume of air left in lungs after maximal exhalation (cannot be expired) NB: not measured by spirometry

(Continued)

(Continued)

Measurement	Normal value	Calculation	Details
Expiratory reserve volume (ERV)	1.2 L	(Spirometry)	Volume of extra air that can be expired at the end of normal breath out
Inspiratory reserve volume (IRV)	3.6 L	(Spirometry) VC – (TV + ERV)	Volume of extra air that can be inhaled at the end of a normal breath in
Functional residual capacity (FRC)	2.4 L	ERV + RV	Volume of air left in lungs at the end of a normal breath out
Inspiratory capacity (IC)	4.1 L	TV + IRV	Volume of air that can be inhaled after a normal breath out
Anatomical dead space (V_T)	150 mL	(Spirometry)	Total volume of conducting airways
Physiological dead space (V_D)	155 mL	$VT \times \dfrac{P_A CO_2 - P_E CO_2}{P_A CO_2}$	Anatomical dead space and alveolar dead space

NB: Dead space is inhaled air that does not take part in gas exchange. Anatomical dead space is the gas in the conducting areas of the respiratory system (e.g. mouth, trachea) that does not come into contact with the alveoli.

Flow-volume loops

Flow-volume loops provide a graphical illustration of a patient's spirometric efforts. Flow is plotted against volume to display a continuous loop from inspiration to expiration.

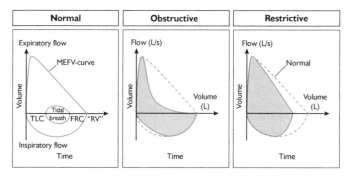

Figure 3.6: Flow volume loops

Acid-base balance

This can be a complex topic. While going into the fundamentals of physiology is beyond the scope of this chapter, understanding a few basic principles can greatly assist in interpreting what is an important investigation – the arterial blood gas. Essentially, analysis of the acid-base balance should determine the size and the direction of the change, which should then be further interpreted in the clinical context.

Henderson–Hasselbalch equation

■ Buffer solutions are able to maintain a constant pH despite the addition of small amounts of acid or base.

■ Such 'classic' buffers are solutions of a weak acid and a conjugated base. Any small amounts of acid or base that are added are absorbed by the buffer solution.

■ The pH of these buffer solutions can be calculated using the Henderson-Hasselbalch equation – a formula to quantify the relationship between [H$^+$], [HCO$_3^-$] and PCO$_2$:

$$pH = pK_a + \log_{10}\frac{[base]}{[acid]}$$

■ The equation describes the derivation of pH as a measure of acidity (using pK$_a$, the acid dissociation constant) and, in addition to estimating the pH of buffer solutions, can also be used to estimate charges on ionisable species in solution (such as amino acid side chains in proteins) and to find the equilibrium pH of acid-base reactions.

■ 'Base' represents the conjugate base and 'acid' the conjugate acid (of a conjugate acid–base pair).

■ The equation assumes that the concentration of the acid and its conjugate base at equilibrium will remain the same as the 'main' concentration.

■ As the dissociation of the acid, the hydrolysis of the base and the dissociation of water itself is ignored, the equation will not work with relatively strong acids or bases.

Anion gap

What is the anion gap?

■ It represents the concentration of the unmeasured anions in the plasma.

■ Sodium (Na$^+$) and potassium (K$^+$) are the predominant positively charged ions (cations).

■ Chloride (Cl$^-$) and bicarbonate (HCO$_3^-$) are the predominant negatively charged molecules (anions).

Hence, the gap is the difference between these.

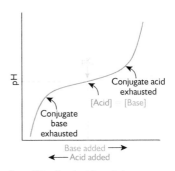

Figure 3.7: pH and acid-base balance

When is it used?

■ The anion gap is used to identify the type of metabolic acidosis to help in differentiating between the various causes (high anion gap versus normal anion gap metabolic acidosis).

■ Normal gap: in an 'inorganic' metabolic acidosis (e.g. due to acid (HCl) infusion), the infused Cl^- replaces HCO_3^- and the anion gap remains normal.

■ Increased gap: in an 'organic' acidosis, the lost bicarbonate is replaced by the acid anion which is not normally measured. This means that the gap is increased.

$$Anion\ gap = (Na^+ + K^+)$$
$$- (Cl^- + HCO_3^-)$$
$$e.g.\ 13.5\ mMol/L$$
$$= (140 + 3.5) - (105 + 25)$$

Normal range $= 8{-}16\ mmol/L$

Approach to metabolic acidosis

In a patient with metabolic acidosis, determining the anion gap allows some of the causes to be isolated.

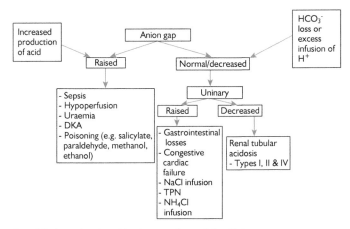

Figure 3.8: Approach to determining the cause of a metabolic acidosis

Arterial blood gas (ABG)

The basics

■ Blood is taken using a (usually) pre-filled heparinised syringe, usually from the radial or femoral arteries. The brachial artery can also be used but this is not common. Prior to taking the sample, the heparin must be expelled from the syringe. Once taken, any surplus air must be expelled from the syringe and the sample analysed promptly.

■ The sample is analysed by a machine that in most hospitals is situated in the emergency or intensive care department. It measures the partial pressure of oxygen (P_aO_2) and carbon dioxide (P_aCO_2), the pH and bicarbonate levels in arterial blood. The base excess (BE), anion gap and the concentrations of sodium (Na^+), potassium (K^+), chloride (Cl-) and lactate can also be measured by some machines.

■ Remember, if a patient is receiving supplemental O_2, this will have to be considered when interpreting the results. Always document the concentration of O_2 being received (FiO_2) on the ABG results printout, as well as the patient details and date/time.

■ Interpreting ABGs is straightforward provided you stick to a few basic rules, work systematically and always consider the results in the context of the clinical situation.

■ Although one-off ABGs can be very useful in certain acute clinical settings, observing trends is also just as important.

Indications

■ Respiratory failure: symptoms and signs of CO_2 retention or hypoxia (to aid diagnosis and to determine severity, e.g. exacerbation of asthma or COPD).

■ Emergency and intensive care monitoring of sick patients (e.g. patients with organ failure, trauma, diabetic ketoacidosis (DKA), burns, sepsis, decreased consciousness, impaired respiratory effort, etc.).

■ To assess ventilation and to aid pH balance.

■ Elective monitoring (during/post surgical procedures, sleep studies).

Oxygen saturation curve

■ Note the sudden fall in PO_2 at a saturation of around 92%.

■ This is why ABGs are usually performed when the saturation drops below this point.

■ After this point, due to the shape of the curve a small drop in O_2 saturation means a large drop in PO_2).

> ✓ **TIP:** Depending on the clinical situation, consider performing an ABG if O_2 saturations drop below 92% (in patients in whom the normal O_2 saturation is above this).

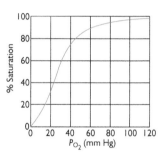

Figure 3.9: Oxygen saturation curve

What are the different aspects of the ABG?

There are five key components of arterial blood to consider.

1 pH
2 Partial pressure of oxygen (P_aO_2)
3 Partial pressure of carbon dioxide (P_aCO_2) – one of the acidic components of blood
(These are measured in kilopascals (KPa) and represent the short-term component of an ABG)

4 Bicarbonate (HCO_3^-) – the alkaline component of blood
5 Base excess (BE)
(These represent the longer-term or compensatory component of the ABG, usually taking at least 24 hours to alter significantly)

Interpreting the ABG

It is important to determine the type of abnormality and for how long it has been present.

1 pH
- Normal = 7.35–7.45
- Acidosis = <7.35
- Alkalosis = >7.45

2 P_aCO_2
- Look at the P_aCO_2 (respiratory) component.
- This tends to change in acute disorders, whereas the HCO_3^- (the metabolic component) is more a long-term compensatory mechanism. If the P_aCO_2 is increased and the pH is low, there is a respiratory acidosis.
- If there is no change in pH, the acidosis has been compensated for.

3 HCO_3^-
- Look at the HCO_3^- (metabolic) component.
- Any changes in HCO_3^- tend to take longer to occur than changes in P_aCO_2.
- Are the pH and bicarbonate low? This indicates metabolic acidosis. Think of the bicarbonate in the blood as being 'used up' to buffer the excess acid.

4 PaO_2
- Look at the PaO_2. Is it normal, increased or low?

- Is the PaO_2 consistent with the amount of O_2 therapy the patient is receiving (FiO_2)? A higher inspired concentration of O_2 should mean a higher PaO_2.
- With an inspired O_2 concentration of 28%, a P_aO_2 of 21 kPa is expected, whereas with 100% O_2, a PaO_2 of 89 kPa would be expected (in theory). Therefore, if the patient has a P_aO_2 of 15 kPa but is receiving 60% oxygen, alarm bells should ring and further investigation into the perfusion status may be warranted.
- In general, a low PaO_2 indicates respiratory failure (V/Q mismatch) and additional respiratory support (e.g. O_2) may be required.

Inspired O_2	Expected PaO_2
28%	21 kPa
40%	32 kPa
60%	51 kPa
100%	89 kPa

5 Base excess
- Look at the base excess.
- Simple: this is effectively the amount of base in the blood. It is usually kept within strict limits and is a sensitive measure of acidosis/alkalosis.
- Complex: quantity of acid or base necessary to titrate 1 litre of blood to pH 7.4 at 37°C with a $PaCO_2$ of 5.3 kPa.

If base excess is >2, there is too much base in the blood (alkalosis)
If base excess is <2, there is too little base in the blood (acidosis)

6 Anion gap

■ Lastly, if necessary (for example in patients with metabolic acidosis), look at the anion gap. The machine may not always calculate this so you will have to do it yourself *(see the section above on how to do this)*.

■ An increased anion gap could be due to DKA, lactic acidosis and aspirin/metformin overdose *(see table below)*.

mmHg to kPa conversion tip
To convert pressure in mmHg to kPa, divide the value in mmHg by 7.5

Table of combinations
The table below shows a range of different combinations of pH, PaCO$_2$.

'Actual' pH	Direction of compensatory pH	PaCO$_2$	BE	Description
N	–	N	0	Normal status
↑	–	↓	0	Acute respiratory alkalosis
↑	↓	↓	–ve	Chronic respiratory alkalosis (with metabolic compensation)
↑	↓	↑	+ve	Non-respiratory alkalosis (with a degree of respiratory compensation)
↓	–	↑	0	Acute respiratory acidosis
↓	↑	↑	+ve	Chronic respiratory acidosis (with metabolic compensation)
↓	↑	↓	–ve	Metabolic acidosis (with respiratory compensation)
↓	–	N	–ve	Metabolic acidosis
N	↑	↓	–ve	Metabolic acidosis (with complete compensation)
↓	–	↑	–ve	Mixed respiratory and metabolic acidosis
↑	–	↓	+ve	Mixed respiratory and metabolic alkalosis

Key: N = normal
NB: 'Compensated' acidosis/alkalosis = underlying acidosis/alkalosis, but the pH of the blood has been returned to normal by compensatory mechanisms.

pH/HCO₃⁻ nomograms

Plotting the pH and HCO₃⁻ changes can be helpful in determining the type of change that has occurred in the pH balance.

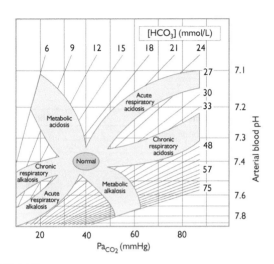

Figure 3.10: Acid-base nomogram

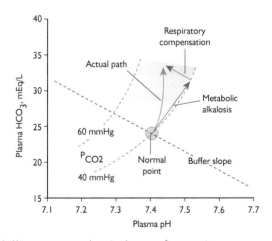

Figure 3.11: Using a nomogram to determine the nature of compensation

Normal values

These are example values for normal healthy patients breathing room air (21% O_2). Please note that normal range values can vary between individuals.

pH	7.35–7.45
P_aO_2	>10.6 kPa (75–100 mmHg)
P_aCO_2	4.7–6.0 kPa (35–45 mmHg)
HCO_3^-	22–28 mmol/L
Base excess	+/–2 mmol/L

Causes of acid-base disturbance

	Acidosis	Alkalosis
Metabolic	*Raised anion gap* **M**ethanol **U**raemia **D**iabetic ketoacidosis (DKA) **P**araldehyde **I**ron tablets/**I**soniazid **L**actic acidosis (common) **E**toH (alcohol)/ethylene glycol **S**alicylates *Normal anion gap* – Diarrhoea (gut HCO_3^- loss) – Renal tubular acidosis	Vomiting Diarrhoea Antacids Hyperaldosteronism (Hypokalaemia)
Respiratory	Respiratory failure – Acute disease (pulmonary embolus, pneumothorax, severe and life-threatening asthma) – Chronic disease (COPD) – CNS depression (opioids, sedatives) – Neuromuscular weakness (Guillain Barré, poliomyelitis)	Hyperventilation (acute asthma attack, panic attack, sepsis, stroke) Early salicylate overdose

Respiratory failure

This is a state of inadequate ventilation. There are two main types.

■ Type 1 = 1 abnormality:
• low PO_2 (<8 kPa)
• normal/low PCO_2 (usually a V/Q mismatch).

■ Type 2 = 2 abnormality:
• low PO_2
• high PCO_2 (with or without V/Q mismatch)
• caused by alveolar hypoventilation.

Note that the classification below can be misleading at times (for example, asthma causes type 1 respiratory failure before it causes type 2).

Examples of causes

Type I	Type II
Atelectasis	Central nervous system (CNS) depression (drugs, sleep, head injury)
Pulmonary oedema – cardiogenic and non-cardiogenic (acute respiratory distress syndrome, ARDS)	Neuromuscular disorders (high spinal cord lesions, poliomyelitis, Guillain-Barré, phrenic nerve lesions)
Infection (pneumonia)	Thoracic wall disease (severe kyphoscoliosis)
Pleural effusion	Pulmonary disease (asthma/COPD/pneumonia). NB: asthma causes type 1 before type 2 failure
Haemo or pneumothorax	Any type I causes (when in an advanced state)
Pulmonary embolus	
Asthma/emphysema	
Pulmonary fibrosis (fibrosing alveolitis)	

Alveolar-arterial (A-a) gradient calculation

The basics

■ This is the difference in O_2 partial pressures between the alveolar and arterial circulations.

■ Calculating the value can help determine if the hypoventilation in type II respiratory failure is due to lung disease or poor respiratory effort (i.e. the cause of hypoxaemia).

A = alveolar / a = arterial

R = respiratory quotient (≈ 0.8) → rises if increased carbohydrates in diet, lower if increased lipids

PB = barometric pressure (≈ 101 kPa at sea level)

PH_2O = water saturation of inspired gas (≈ 6.2 k Pa) → fully saturated

FiO_2 = fractional concentration of O_2 in inspired air (e.g. 0.21 with room air which contains 21% O_2)

$$(A\text{-}a)PO_2 = PAO_2 - PaO_2$$

Normal range = 0.2–1.5 kPa (room air)
(NB: this increases with age → 1.5–3 kPa (75 years))

$$PAO_2 = (PB - PH_2O) \times FiO_2 - \frac{PaCO_2}{R}$$
$$= (101 - 6.2) \times 0.21 - \frac{8.}{0.8}$$
$$= 10 \text{ kPa (breathing room air and with a } PaCO_2 \text{ of 8 kPa)}$$

Pneumonia severity

A simple way in which to determine the severity and subsequently the prognosis of pneumonia, is to calculate the British Thoracic Society's 'CURB-65' score of adverse features:

C – **C**onfusion (AMTS ≤8)
U – **U**rea (>7 mmol/L)
R – **R**espiratory rate (≥30/min)
B – **B**P (systolic <90 mmHg and/or <60 mmHg diastolic)
65 – age >65

Score

Each positive feature = 1 point. A score >1 suggests severe disease.

Prognosis

Score	%mortality
1	0
2	3.2
3	17
4	41
5	57

Pleural effusion

These are excess collections of fluid that accumulate in the pleural space. It is useful to categorise the type of effusion based on the protein concentration to help determine the cause of the effusion. This can be achieved by aspirating a small sample of the pleural fluid (pleural tap). The key distinguishing features are discussed in the table below.

Transudate versus exudates

	Transudate	Exudate
Protein	<25 g/L	>35 g/L
Protein (pleural fluid:serum ratio)	<0.5	>0.5
Lactate dehydrogenase (LDH) (pleural fluid:serum ratio)	<0.6	>0.6 (>2/3 normal limit for serum)
Site	Often bilateral	Often unilateral
Causes	Heart (left ventricular) failure, liver hepatic cirrhosis (liver failure) and other hypoalbuminamic states, renal failure	Infection (e.g. pneumonia/tuberculosis), malignancy, pulmonary embolus, pancreatitis, rheumatoid arthritis

Other features of the fluid that can aid diagnosis include the following.

■ Colour:
• straw (like apple juice or clear urine) = normal
• white/chylous (chylothorax) = lymph
• turbid and yellow = infection
• bloody (haemothorax = frank blood) = trauma, pulmonary embolus, malignancy.
■ pH:
• e.g. low (acidic) in infection (empyaema).
■ Staining/culture:

- e.g. Ziehl-Nielson acid-fast staining for tuberculosis.
■ Cytology:
- differential cell count suggests nature of infection (e.g. bacterial versus viral)
- can detect malignant cells.
■ Autoantibody screen:
- e.g. rheumatoid factor suggests rheumatoid arthritis, while anti-nuclear antibody (ANA) suggests systemic lupus erythematosus (SLE).
■ Glucose:
- can be low in rheumatoid arthritis.
■ Enzymes:
- e.g. amylase = high in pancreatitis (secondary pleural effusion).

Pulmonary embolus (PE)

Assessing the probability of PE

■ The British Thoracic Society has concluded that scoring systems to clas-

sify PE into 'likely' and 'unlikely' are either inaccurate or too complex for practical use.
■ However, such systems are often favoured by hospitals as they provide a quantitative approach to risk stratification. A simple system of assessing clinical probability in patients with possible PE asks two questions.
■ Is another diagnosis unlikely (chest radiograph and ECG are helpful)?
■ Is there a major risk factor (recent immobility/major surgery/lower limb trauma or surgery, pregnancy/post partum, major medical illness, previous proven venous thromboembolism)?
Low = neither; Intermediate = either; High = both.
  More in-depth assessment of probability can be undertaken by use of the methods below.

Wells' score

Active cancer with ongoing treatment or treatment within the previous 6 months or palliative care	1 point
Paralysis, paresis or recent immobilisation of the legs in plaster	1 point
Recently confined to bed for more than 3 days or major surgery within 4 weeks	1 point
Localised tenderness along the distribution of the deep venous system	1 point
Whole leg swollen	1 point
Calf swelling by more than 3 cm compared with the asymptomatic leg (measured 10 cm below the tibial tuberosity)	1 point
Pitting oedema more marked in the symptomatic leg	1 point
Collateral superficial veins, not varicose veins	1 point
Alternative diagnosis as likely or more likely than DVT	−2 points

Score: 0 = low probability, 1 or 2 = moderate probability, 3 or more = high probability.

Risk factors for venous thromboembolism (VTE)

(Taken from BTS Guidelines for the management of suspected acute pulmonary embolism. Thorax 2003; 58: 470–84)

Major risk factors (relative risk 5–20)	
Surgery*	■ Major abdominal/pelvic surgery ■ Hip/knee replacement ■ Postoperative intensive care
Obstetrics	■ Late pregnancy ■ Caesarian section ■ Puerperium
Lower limb problems	■ Fracture ■ Varicose veins
Malignancy	■ Abdominal/pelvic ■ Advanced/metastatic
Reduced mobility	■ Hospitalisation ■ Institutional care
Miscellaneous	■ Previous proven VTE
Minor risk factors (relative risk 2–4)	
Cardiovascular	■ Congenital heart disease ■ Congestive cardiac failure ■ Hypertension ■ Superficial venous thrombosis ■ Indwelling central vein catheter
Oestrogens	■ Oral contraceptive ■ Hormone replacement therapy
Miscellaneous	■ COPD ■ Neurological disability ■ Occult malignancy ■ Thrombotic disorders ■ Long-distance sedentary travel ■ Obesity ■ Other†

*Where appropriate prophylaxis is used, relative risk is much lower.
†Inflammatory bowel disease, nephrotic syndrome, chronic dialysis, myeloproliferative disorders.

Pulmonary fibrosis

Causes of apical fibrosis

Extrinsic allergic alveolitis
Sarcoid
Coal workers pneumoconiosis
Histiocytosis X (now known as Langerhans cell histiocytosis)
Ankylosing spondylitis
Tuberculosis

Causes of basal fibrosis

Rheumatoid arthritis
Asbestosis
Scleroderma
Cryptogenic fibrosing alveolitis (also known as 'idiopathic pulmonary fibrosis', with the histological pattern described as UIP – Usual Interstitial Pneumonitis)
Other (drugs, e.g. bleomycin, nitrofurantoin, amiodarone)

Tumours of the lung

Primary

■ Lung tumours (primary and secondary) are the commonest type of malignancy in the world.
■ Primary lung tumours include: small-cell, adenocarcinoma (NSCLC, non-small cell lung carcinoma), squamous cell carcinoma (NSCLC) and large-cell.
■ Cytology of sputum and pleural fluid is a useful investigation to evaluate the presence of malignancy.
■ Definitive diagnosis of the different types of malignancy requires samples for histological analysis.

Secondary (metastasis)

■ These are common and can follow three common patterns:
• miliary
• cannonball (single large spherical tumour)
• lymphangitis carcinomatosis (lymphatic spread).
■ Histologically, they can show features typical of their tissue of origin.

■ Commonly originate from **B**reast, **L**ung, **T**hyroid, **K**idneys, **P**rostate.
■ Mnemonic: BLT-KP (think of a Bacon Lettuce & Tomato sandwich with Ketchup & Pickles).

Other tests

There are several other investigations that can be useful in investigating respiratory disease. These include the following.

Urine
■ *Legionella pneumophila* antigen test: blood cultures can have a broad range of sensitivities, therefore urinary assays (e.g. by an enzyme-linked immunosorbant assay, ELISA) can help confirm a diagnosis.

Sputum/Pleural fluid
■ Sputum samples can be easily obtained for cytology and microscopy, culture and antibiotic sensitivities (M, C & S).
■ These are useful in the diagnosis of conditions such as malignancy and tuberculosis.

Skin
■ Tuberculin test: used in the investigation of tuberculosis. Positive results (a lymphocyte mediated type 4 hypersensitivity reaction) can suggest active, recent or past infection, and can also occur after immunisation.
■ Mantoux test: serial dilutions provide different titres of TB antigen. Controvertial test, but broadly regarded as positive if ≥10 mm induration, and negative if <5 mm.
■ Sweat test: used in the investigation of cystic fibrosis (raised concentrations of

sodium and chloride are present – the guidelines indicate a sweat chloride concentration of >60 mmol/L is consistent with a diagnosis of cystic fibrosis).

Blood

■ Alpha-1 antitrypsin: deficiency of this enzyme can lead to pan-acinar emphysema.

■ Serology/complement fixation: these tests can be used to investigate viral pneumonia (e.g. cause by *Mycoplasma pneumonia* or *Legionella pneumonia*).

■ IgE/eosinophil count: useful in the investigation of atopic disease (e.g. asthma).

Imaging

■ A number of imaging modalities can be particularly helpful in the diagnosis of respiratory conditions.

■ These include chest x-ray (CXR) and computed tomography (CT), as well as other specialist variations e.g. high resolution spiral CT and positron emission tomography (PET) CT, and wider imaging modalities, including bone scanning.

■ Please see Chapter 15 for more details.

Endoscopy

■ Bronchoscopy: this involves either a rigid or flexible instrument to visualise the bronchial tree. This can be of use in the investigation of bronchial malignancy or certain infections (e.g. *Pneumocystis jirovecii*). Samples can be taken by broncho-alveolar lavage/washings, which can then be examined by microscopy, cytology or culture.

Lung biopsy

■ This involves removal and analysis of a piece of lung tissue.

■ Biopsy can be either bronchoscopy based, needle based (percutaneous, usually with image guidance), open (e.g. during surgery) or video-assisted (with the assistance of a thoracoscope).

■ It is used in the histological diagnosis of certain conditions, such as pulmonary fibrosis or sarcoidosis. Cytological examination of the biopsy specimen can also be of use in the investigation of malignancy.

Overnight sleep studies (polysomnography)

■ These are used to assess sleep patterns as well as the body functions during sleep.

■ This usually involves monitoring of various parameters during sleep, including eye movements (electrooculography, EOG), brain activity (electroencephalogram, EEG), cardiac activity (electrocardiogram, ECG) and muscle activity (electromyelogram, EMG) as well as respiratory effort/function (e.g. pulse oxymetry).

■ These can be supplemented by other measures such as body temperature and penile tumescence, etc.

■ This can be useful in the investigation of conditions such as obstructive sleep apnoea syndrome.

■ Chapter 7 contains more details regarding some of these investigations (e.g. EEG, EMG, etc.).

Chapter 4
GASTROENTEROLOGY

Introduction

Gastroenterological investigations encompass the gastrointestinal tract (from mouth to anus), as well as the hepato-biliary system (liver, gall bladder, pancreas). Although a detailed history may be very helpful, clinical examination can often yield non-specific findings. This places greater importance on the use of appropriate investigations to help facilitate diagnosis and aid subsequent management. Remember that imaging (in the form of x-ray, CT/MRI, contrast studies, etc.) is often a very helpful adjunct. While this chapter discusses some of the more specialty-specific techniques, the application of more 'standard' modalities to gastrointestinal imaging is considered further in Chapter 15.

Topics covered
- General investigations
- *Helicobacter pylori*
- Endoscopy
- Inflammatory bowel disease (IBD)
- Autoimmune gut disease
- Gastrointestinal (GI) bleed
- Jaundice
- Liver function tests (LFTs)
- Autoimmune liver and biliary tract disease
- Hepatitis
- Ascites
- Severity of liver disease: Child-Pugh classification
- Liver decompensation
- Paracetamol poisoning
- Indications for liver transplant
- Pancreatitis
- Nutrition
- Histological findings in GI disease

NB: Please note that any 'normal ranges' quoted may vary between individuals and laboratories.

General investigations

Blood tests

- A number of 'routine' blood tests can be of use when investigating gastrointestinal pathology, e.g. full blood count (e.g. anaemias), urea and electrolytes (e.g. diarrhoeas).
- Liver function tests: of particular use in hepato-biliary pathologies. These are considered in more detail later in this chapter.
- Other relevant biochemical tests: include haematinics (iron studies, e.g. in haemochromatosis) and copper/caeruloplasmin (e.g. in Wilson's disease).

The hands-on guide to data interpretation. By S. Abraham, K. Kulkarni, R. Madhu and D. Provan. Published 2010 by Blackwell Publishing Ltd.

■ Viral serology: particularly important when considering viral hepatitis. The different agents responsible for viral hepatitis are considered in more detail later.

■ Autoimmune antibodies: a number of antibodies play a role in autoimmune gastrointestinal disease, including anti-mitochondrial antibody, anti-smooth muscle antibody, anti-nuclear factor.

■ Other blood tests: these include serum gastrin (gastrinoma, Zollinger-Ellison syndrome), and various tumour markers (e.g. alpha-fetoprotein for hepatocellular carcinoma, carcinoembryonic antigen for colonic cancer).

Imaging

■ A number of imaging techniques can be helpful when investigating gastrointestinal pathology. These include:

• plain abdominal x-ray (e.g. bowel obstruction, inflammatory bowel disease)

• ultrasound (e.g. biliary tract stones)

• CT (e.g. malignancy)

• barium/gastrograffin (contrast) studies (e.g. inflammatory bowel disease).

See Chapter 15 for more details of these.

Liver biopsy

■ This is usually image-guided (e.g. by ultrasound/CT) and plays an important management and prognostic role in conditions such as chronic hepatitis and cirrhosis.

See Chapter 15 for more details of these.

pH

■ This is useful in the investigation of gastro-oesophageal reflux.

■ Measurement is often undertaken over 24 h.

■ Positive tests = more than one event of reflux (pH <4) per hour. Broadly speaking, a pH <4 should be present for no more than 10.5% (erect) or 6% (supine) of the time.

Manometry

■ Measurement of oesophageal pressures is useful in the investigation of 'non-cardiac' chest pain, dysphagia/gastro-oesophageal reflux disease (GORD) and other oesophageal disorders such as achalasia.

■ Achalasia is associated with a general lack of oesophageal motility and failure of relaxation of the lower oesophageal sphincter.

NB: The pressures of other GI sphincters can also be recorded using similar techniques (e.g. anal sphincter).

Stool tests

The composition of stool can often yield valuable information about the function of the gastrointestinal tract. Appearance alone can be useful.

■ Dark 'tarry' black (with a characteristic odour) = melaena (contains digested blood).

■ Pale = obstructive jaundice (e.g. secondary to gallstones) or malabsorption (steatorrhoea – especially if stools are floaty and difficult to flush, as there is a higher fat content due to impaired pancreatic enzyme function).

Other stool investigations that can be undertaken, include the following.

■ Culture.

■ Microscopy: for ova, cysts and parasites (e.g. Giardia lamblia, Entamoeba histolytica).

■ Faecal occult blood (FOB): used for detecting quantities of blood in stool that are not adequate to be visualised. FOB testing has poor–moderate sensitivity and specificity in individuals, but is useful in population screening. Newer versions using immuno-staining appear more sensitive/specific but have not yet reached widespread use.

■ Fat and elastase: these tests are useful in patients with suspected malabsorption, e.g. due to pancreatic insufficiency or bacterial overgrowth.

Bristol Stool Chart (Meyers Scale)

■ Used to classify faeces into different categories. This can assist in defining a patient's symptoms.

■ The shape and texture of the stool depends on the time it spends in the colon.

■ In general, 1 and 2 suggest constipation, 3 and 4 are 'normal' and 5–7 suggest diarrhoea/ urgency.

Bristol stool chart	
Type 1	Separate hard lumps like nuts (hard to pass)
Type 2	Sausage-shaped but lumpy
Type 3	Like a sausage but with cracks on its surface
Type 4	Like a sausage or snake, smooth and soft
Type 5	Soft blobs with clear-cut edges (passed easily)
Type 6	Fluffy pieces with ragged edges, a mushy stool
Type 7	Watery, no solid pieces. Entirely liquid

Figure 4.1: Bristol Stool Chart. Source: Lewis SJ, Heaton KW (1997). Stool form scale as a useful guide to intestinal transit time. Scand. J. Gastroenterol. 32(9): 920–4.

Helicobacter pylori (H. pylori)

■ This gram negative, microaerophilic bacterium is found in the upper gastrointestinal tract (stomach and duodenum).

■ Although many people are asymptomatic to *H. pylori* colonisation, it is a common cause of peptic ulcer disease. Diagnosis and subsequent eradiation is therefore of importance in the treatment of ulcers and dyspeptic symptoms.

■ Eradication is classically by 'triple therapy': LAC (lansoprazole, amoxicillin and clarithromycin) or LAM (lansoprazole, amoxicillin and metronidazole).

■ There are several different investigations available.

Breath tests

■ Non-invasive.

■ *H. pylori* produces urease via the breakdown of urea to form ammonia and CO_2.

■ Patient is given a tablet containing ^{13}C Urea (radio-labelled).

■ If *H. pylori* is present, $^{13}CO_2$ (radio-labelled CO_2) is produced and detected in the breath.

Campylobacter-like organism (CLO) test

■ Considered the most sensitive standard (i.e. widely available/non-research) test.

■ Invasive.

■ Biopsy samples (taken at oesophagealgastroduodenoscopy, OGD) are placed into a medium containing urea and phenol red.

■ If *H. pylori* is present, ammonia will be liberated from the urea in the medium.

■ Phenol red produces a red colour in alkaline solutions, hence the presence of *H. pylori* and the release of ammonia will cause the medium to turn red.

■ Note that this test may be less sensitive in certain situations, e.g. when patients are using proton pump inhibitors.

Other investigations

■ *H. pylori* direct IgG antibody detection (false positives for 1 year post-eradication).

■ Tissue biopsy: microscopy (histological specimen analysis) and culture for *H. pylori*.

Endoscopy

■ Fibreoptic endoscopy is commonly used to visualise the gastrointestinal (GI) tract.

■ In addition, endoscopy allows biopsy samples to be taken for histological study.

■ With the ability to, for example, remove small masses of tissues (e.g. polyps), this can be considered both, an investigative and a therapeutic tool.

Oesophagogastroduo-denoscopy (OGD)

■ This is endoscopy of the upper GI tract.

■ It can help visualise pathology from the oesophagus through to the duodenum, e.g. gastric malignancy, peptic ulcer disease, varices, etc.

■ Also useful as a therapeutic tool, for example to help manage GI bleeds.

■ OGD reports contain written descriptions of the findings at each of the three regions (oesophagus, stomach, duodenum), often accompanied by photographs of any pathology noted.

■ Complications include those related to sedation, perforation and aspiration.

Endoscopic retrograde cholangio-pancreatography (ERCP)

■ This combines the use of a side-viewing endoscope with a contrast medium and radiological imaging.

■ Its primary use is in visualising biliary tract, for example in the investigation of stones or malignancy.

■ The ERCP scope can also be used to cut (cutting/sphincterotomy is not done with the scope but with an accessory that has a cutting wire (sphincterotomy – to allow stones to pass more freely), to pass stents and to directly relieve stones with a balloon.

■ Complications include those related to sedation, pancreatitis and cholangitis (perforation and bleeding).

Sigmoidoscopy

■ This is used to visualise part of the lower GI tract (only the left colon).

■ It can help visualise pathologies of the anus, rectum and large bowel, e.g. malignancies, polyps, distal colitis.

■ There are two types:

• Rigid: this rigid (fixed shape) instrument is approximately 25 cm long and can visualise up to the rectum.

• Flexible: this flexible instrument is approximately 60 cm long and can visualise up to the splenic flexure. A pre-procedure enema is often performed. This is usually performed without sedation.

Colonoscopy

■ This flexible instrument is approximately 180 cm long and allows the entire large bowel to be visualised. This is usually about as far proximal as the colonoscope goes (this goes into the terminal ileum).

■ Bowel preparation with enemas/laxatives is used in advance, and sedation is almost always used.

■ Complications include those related to sedation, haemorrhage and perforation (the latter two are more likely to occur if a biopsy has been taken or polyps have been resected).

Inflammatory bowel disease

In the context of data interpretation, inflammatory bowel disease is likely to be encountered in a variety of investigation reports. These include endoscopic findings (e.g. colonoscopy, rigid and flexible sigmoidoscopy), the subsequent histological reports (of biopsy samples taken at endoscopy), contrast studies and imaging (plain X-ray, CT, MRI).

Key differences between Crohn's disease and ulcerative colitis (UC)

	Crohn's disease	Ulcerative colitis
Site	Affects any part of the gastrointestinal tract from mouth to anus	Starts at rectum and 'spreads' proximally. Limited to the large intestine
Macroscopic/ Imaging features	Patchy, full-thickness inflammation ('cobblestone mucosa'), with islands of normal mucosa in between (skips lesions) and rose thorn ulcers	Superficial inflammation (confined to mucosa) with pseudopolyps
Histological features	Transmural inflammation Non-caseating granulomas Fissuring ulcers Lymphoid aggregates Neutrophil infiltrates	Mucosal and submucosa involvement Mucosal ulcers Inflammatory cell infiltrate Crypt abscesses Loss of goblet cells
Perianal disease	Significant perianal disease (abscess/fistulae, etc) present in 25–35% of cases.	No significant perianal disease
Fistulating disease	Fistulae are common	Fistulae do not occur

Truelove-Witts criteria: categorising the severity of ulcerative colitis

Assessing disease severity is important in both management and determining prognosis. The Truelove-Witts criteria is a useful system for stratifying the severity of UC disease.

The mnemonic 'H PEST' is a good way of remembering the categories.

		Mild	Severe
H	Haemoglobin (Hb)	>10 g/dL (i.e. normal)	≤10.5 g/dL or <75% of normal
P	Pulse rate	<90/min	≥90/min
E	ESR	<30 mm/h	≥30 mm/h
S	Stool frequency	≤4 bowel movements/day	>6 bowel movements/day
T	Temperature	<37.5°C (i.e. apyrexial)	≥37.8°C

NB: Intermediate disease = features in between the above two categories.

Crohn's Disease Activity Index (CDAI)

■ This is a research tool used to quantify the severity of the symptoms of an episode of Crohn's disease.

■ It is helpful when assessing the efficacy of treatments. It consists of six factors, adjusted by a weighting factor. One point is added for each of the complications

Clinical or laboratory variable	Weighting factor
1 Number of liquid or soft stools each day for 7 days	x2
2 Abdominal pain (graded 0–3 on severity) each day for 7 days	x5
3 General wellbeing, subjectively assessed from 0 (well) to 4 (terrible) each day for 7 days	x7
4 Presence of complications (e.g. arthralgia, pyrexia, fissures, etc.)	x20
5 Taking co-phenotrope or opiates for diarrhoea	x30
6 Presence of an abdominal mass (0 = none, 2 = questionable, 5 = definite)	x10
7 Absolute deviation of haematocrit from 47% in men and 42% in women	x6
8 Percentage deviation from standard weight	x1

Autoimmune gut disease

Coeliac disease

■ Coeliac disease, an autoimmune phenomenon, is usually triggered by ingested gluten (gliadin), which leads to an immune response to the target auto-antigen tissue transglutaminase (tTG).

■ In addition to this, several other bio-chemical markers that are suggestive of the disease can be found on serum assays.

Antibodies

■ anti-human tissue transglutaminase (tTG) antibody (IgA).

■ IgA or IgG anti-gliadin antibodies (AGA).

■ anti-reticulin antibody (ARA).

■ IgA anti-endomysial antibodies (EmA).

Others

■ Total serum IgA.

■ Genetic testing: HLA-DQ2 and HLA-DQ8.

Gastrointestinal (GI) bleed

■ The Rockall score is a widely used scoring system based on admission and post-endoscopy scores.

■ It can be used to classify the severity of a GI bleed and has been validated for predicting the risk of re-bleeding as well as mortality.

■ Maximum pre-endoscopy score = 7

■ Maximum post-endoscopy score (post-diagnosis) = 11

Rockall score: GI bleed risk classification

Variable	Score			
	0	1	2	3
Age (years)	<60	60–79	>79	–
Shock	BP >100 mmHg	BP>100 mmHg	BP<100 mmHg	–
	Pulse <100	Pulse >100	Pulse >100	
Comorbidity	None	–	Cardiac disease, any other major comorbidity	Renal failure, liver failure, disseminated malignancy
Endoscopic diagnosis	Mallory-Weiss tear, no lesion	All other diagnoses	Malignancy of the upper GI tract	–
Major SRH	None, or dark spots	–	Blood in the upper GI tract, adherent clot or spurting vessel	–

SRH = stigmata of recent haemorrhage.

From the Rockall scoring table, the risk of both rebleeding and mortality can be predicted.

Rebleed/mortality		
Risk score	**Predicted rebleed (%)**	**Predicted mortality (%)**
0	5	0
1	3	0
2	5	0
3	11	3
4	14	5
5	24	11
6	33	17
7	44	27
8+	42	41

Jaundice

■ Jaundice (icterus) is the yellowish discoloration of the skin, conjunctiva (covering of the sclera) and mucous membranes caused by hyperbilirubinaemia and subsequent deposition of bilirubin in the extravascular spaces.

■ This usually occurs when plasma concentrations of bilirubin are approximately >40 μmol/L.

■ The different types of jaundice can be understood by considering the underlying pathways.

• Pre-hepatic: haem (from the haemoglobin of old red blood cells) is oxidised to form biliverdin and the iron attached to the haem is released. Biliverdin is then converted to 'unconjugated' bilirubin. This happens in the intravascular compartment, hence anything that increases the rate of haemolysis can cause pre-hepatic jaundice.

• Hepatic: the unsoluble unconjugated bilirubin then travels to the liver bound to albumin. Catalysed by the enzyme UDP-glucuronide transferase, it is conjugated with glucuronic acid to form soluble bilirubin diglucuronide ('conjugated' bilirubin).

• Post-hepatic: this conjugated bilirubin is excreted from the liver into the biliary and cystic ducts as part of bile. Intestinal bacteria convert it to urobilinogen. This can either be converted to stercobilinogen (oxidised to stercobilin and passed out in the faeces) or it can be reabsorbed by the gut, transported to the kidneys and passed out in the urine (as urobilin). Broadly speaking, post-hepatic jaundice occurs when there is an obstructive problem.

■ Jaundice can therefore occur due to pathologies at any of these three stages, each with its own characteristic features.

Type	Examples	Bilirubin	Urine	Stools
Pre-hepatic	(Autoimmune) haemolysis, Gilbert's and Crigler-Najaar syndromes	Unconjugated	Normal (no bilirubin, urobilinogen+++)	Normal
Hepatic	Hepatitis (infective, drugs, autoimmune)	Mixed	Variable	Variable
Post-hepatic	Gallstones (cholestatic), Dubin-Johnson and Rotor syndromes	Conjugated	Dark (bilirubin+++, no urobilinogen as blocked enterohepatic circulation)	Pale

Liver function tests (LFTs)

Normal range: AST: 1–31 U/L, ALT: 5–35 U/L

These are a collection of blood assays for various liver enzymes and bilirubin. Clotting and albumin are often regarded as the best indicators of 'synthetic' liver function. The clotting cascade are discussed in Chapter 8. Please note, that as with all 'normal ranges', levels can vary between healthy individuals and between different laboratories.

Aminotransferases

■ Aspartate aminotransferase (AST) and alanine aminotransferase (ALT) are the most specific markers of hepatocellular injury and necrosis.
■ AST and ALT catalyse transfer of the alpha-amino groups aspartate and alanine to the alpha-keto group of alpha-ketoglutaric acid.
■ AST = present in a wide variety of tissues (including heart, skeletal muscle, kidney, brain, and liver). ALT = more liver specific.

Alkaline phosphatase (ALP)

■ May originate from bone, liver, intestine, kidney or placenta.
■ In children and adolescents (active bone growth), serum ALP may increase up to 3x.
■ Rise in hepatobiliary disease = increased hepatic production with leakage into the serum rather than from failure to clear or excrete circulating ALP.
■ Marked rise = extrahepatic biliary obstruction, primary biliary cirrhosis, drug-induced cholestasis, primary sclerosing cholangitis and infiltrative processes (e.g. amyloid, granulomatous hepatitis, malignancy).
■ Degree of elevation does not differentiate intra versus extra-hepatic cholestasis.
■ Reduced levels = associated with congenital hypophosphatasia, hypothyroidism, pernicious anaemia and zinc deficiency.

> *Normal range:* 45–105 U/L (over 14 years)

Gamma-glutamyl transferase (GGT)

■ Sensitive indicator of hepatobiliary disease (but not specific). Long T1/2 (26 days).

■ Elevated in renal failure, myocardial infarction, pancreatic disease and diabetes mellitus. Rise also induced by ingestion of phenytoin or alcohol (in the absence of liver disease features).

■ If concomitantly elevated, GGT is useful in excluding a bone source of ALP elevation.

■ Classical role is as a marker of alcohol ingestion and alcoholic liver disease. Isolated elevation with no clinical features of liver disease does not warrant further investigation.

> *Normal range:* 4–35 U/L (<50 U/L in males)

Bilirubin

■ Binds reversibly to albumin and is transported to the liver, where it is conjugated to glucuronic acid and excreted in the bile.

■ Derived primarily from catabolism of red blood cell haem.

■ Normal serum = small levels of unconjugated and no conjugated bilirubin (although some laboratories do measure small levels of conjugated bilirubin too).

■ Conjugated bilirubin = water-soluble, hence excreted in the urine (dark urine in obstructive jaundice).

> *Normal range:* 1–22 µmol/L (total bilirubin)

Albumin

■ This is the most abundant plasma protein.

■ It is responsible for maintaining plasma oncotic pressure and as a carrier protein for non-specifically binding to various substances in the bloodstream.

> *Normal range:* 37–49 g/L

Amylase

■ Although not strictly related to the liver, this enzyme is one that is often checked when investigating abdominal pain.

■ It is released from the pancreas, usually in particularly elevated amounts during acute inflammation (e.g. acute pancreatitis).

■ Amylase is not 100% specific to the pancreas. Other pathologies can also lead to elevated levels (e.g. parotid gland inflammation), mild elevation is non-specific and can occur in other circumstances (e.g. perforated ulcer).

■ Note that in cases of chronic pancreatitis, levels may be relatively normal.

> *Normal range:* 60–180 U/L

Common patterns of raised liver enzymes

NB: Remember that the table below is a rather crude indicator of the aetiology of the liver disease and should always be used in the context of the clinical history and examination. The severity of the particular condition will always affect the extent to which the enzymes are raised.

Test (normal range, IU/L)	AST (11–32)	ALT (3–30)	ALP (35–105)	GGT (2–65)
Hepatocellular disease	++	++	+	
Cholestatic (obstructive)	+	+	+++	+++
Infiltrative disease	N/+	N/+	++	++
Alcoholic disease	+++	++	+	+++
Autoimmune hepatitis	++	++	+	
Viral hepatitis	++++	++++		
Toxic/ischaemic injury	+++++	+++++		
Primary biliary cirrhosis	+	+	++	+

'Hepatocellular' (mainly AST/ALT) versus 'cholestatic' (mainly ALP and GGT)

■ **Chronic hepatitis**: predominantly 'hepatocellular' (although mild cholestasis is common).

■ **Biliary obstruction**: hepatocellular pattern often occurs in the *acute* setting (first five days) but cholestatic pattern later (as AST/ALT normalise in *chronic* obstruction).

Autoimmune liver and biliary tract disease

There are a number of different types of autoimmune disease affecting the liver and the biliary tract, each characterised by the presence of different serum antibody markers.

Autoantibody profiles

Antibody	Antigen	Autoimmune Hepatitis I (AIH1)	Autoimmune Hepatitis 2 (AIH2)	Primary biliary cirrhosis (PBC)	AIH1&PBC overlap disease	Primary sclerosing cholangitis (PSC)
Anti-nuclear antibody (ANA)	Sp 100 (nuclear matrix) Gp 210 (Rim ANA)	+		+	+	+
Anti-neutrophil cytoplasmic antibody (ANCA)						+
Anti-smooth muscle Antibody (ASMA)	Actin, Vimentin, Tubulin	+			+/–	
Liver-Kidney microsomes (LKM1)	Cytochrome P450		+			
Liver cytosolic (LC)	Formimino-transferase cyclodeaminase		+			
Soluble liver antigen (SLA/LP)	UGA suppressor tRNA associated protein	+	+		+	
Anti-mitochondrial antibody (AMA)	Pyruvate dehydrogenase complex			+	+	

NB: While the role of ANA and ANCA are stated as classically associated with PBC and PSC respectively, they are by no means the sole diagnostic factors, as they are not positive in all patients with these conditions (e.g. ANCA is only positive in about 60% of patients with PSC).

■ Causes include infective agents (viruses), toxic effects of drugs and chemicals, alcohol, inherited diseases and autoimmune pathologies.

■ Viral hepatitis is most commonly causes by one of three agents: hepatitis A, B and C virus.

■ Blood tests are important in investigating the viral aetiologies.

Hepatitis

■ Hepatitis is inflammation of the liver.

Hepatitis A virus (HAV) serology

	Total anti-HAV (IgM and IgG)	**IgM Anti-HAV**
Acute hepatitis A	Positive	Positive
Resolved hepatitis A	Positive	Negative
Immunisation	Positive	Negative

Hepatitis B virus (HBV) serology

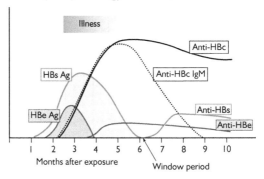

Window period = anti-HBc IgM Ab detectable only

HBsAg = hepatitis B surface antigen (found in cytoplasm of infected hepatocyte)

HBeAg = hepatitis B e antigen (subunit of HBcAg; marker of infectivity as implies viral replication; 'pre-core mutants' exist, which contain no HBe Ag)

HBcAg = hepatitis B core antigen (found in nuclei of infected hepatocytes)

Anti-HBs = hepatitis B surface antibody

Anti-HBe = hepatitis B e antibody

Anti-HBc = hepatitis B core antibody

Figure 4.2: Antibodies in hepatitis B

Time since infection	Stage	HBsAg	Anti-HBs AB	Anti-HBc IgM	Anti-HBc IgG	HbeAg	Anti-Hbe AB	Status
6 weeks–6 months	Incubation period	-	-	-	-	-	-	Not yet infectious
1–2 weeks	Late incubation	++	-	-	-	+ or -	-	Infectious
2–4 weeks	Acute	++	-	++	++	++	-	Infectious
<6 months	HBsAg-negative, still 'acute'	-	-	++	++	-	-	Potentially infectious
6 months–6 years	Recent infection	-	++	+ or -	++	-	++	Infectivity low
Others:								
Infected in (distant) past		-	+	-	+	-	-	Immune (post infection)
Chronic infection		++	-	+ or -	+++	++	-	Infectious
Healthy HBsAg carrier		++	-	+ or -	+++	-	++	Infectious
Immunised		-	+	-	-	-	-	Immune (post immunisation)

AB = antibody

NB: In addition, HBV-DNA can also be assayed on serum samples.

Hepatitis C virus (HCV) serology

Detection test	Anti-HCV AB Enzyme immunoassay (EIA)	Anti-HCV AB Radioimmunoblot assay (RIBA)	HCV RNA Polymerase chain reaction (PCR) or bDNA
Acute	–	–	+
Resolved	+	+	–
Chronic	+	+	+

Ascites

Background

■ Ascites is an excess or abnormal collection of peritoneal fluid in the abdominal cavity.
■ Ascitic fluid samples can be aspirated by abdominal paracentesis (ascitic tap) and sent for analysis to help determine the cause.
■ Like pleural effusions, analysing their constitution can help determine the cause of the ascites.
■ The commonest cause of ascites is portal hypertension secondary to cirrhosis (liver disease).

	Exudate	Transudate
Specific gravity (g/mL)	>1.015	<1.015
Total protein (g/L)	>25	<25
Fluid/serum protein ratio	>0.5	<0.5
Fluid/serum LDH ratio	>0.6	<0.6
Fluid/serum glucose ratio	<1.0 (low glucose can be suggestive of malignancy)	>1.0
Causes	Malignancy, infection (including tuberculosis), pancreatitis, collagen vascular disease, post-pericardiotomy syndrome	Congestive cardiac failure, cirrhosis, nephrotic syndrome, radiation, uraemia, hypothyroidism, trauma

Other features to consider

■ Amylase
• can be raised in pancreatitis.
■ Serum-ascites albumin gradient (g/L) = serum albumin (g/L) − ascitic albumin (g/L)
• if >11 g/L, likely to be portal hypertension.
■ Gram stain, white cell count (WCC), microscopy, culture and sensitivity (M, C & S):
• to detect infection (peritonitis)
• important in patients undergoing peritoneal dialysis, in whom spontaneous bacterial peritonitis (SBP) is a risk
• differential WCC: neutrophils >250 cells/mm^3 = suggestive of SBP
• Gram stain = presence of bacteria

• like blood cultures, ascitic fluid should therefore be sent for M, C & S.
■ Cytology
• to detect malignant cells.

Severity of liver disease: Child-Pugh classification

■ Used to assess the prognosis of chronic liver disease (mainly cirrhosis).
■ This can help determine appropriate management and the need for liver transplantation.
■ The score utilises five clinical measures of liver disease. Each measure is scored 1–3, with 3 indicating the most severe derangement.

	Child-Pugh classification			
Mnemonic	**Clinical or biochemical parameters**	**Points**		
		1	**2**	**3**
A	Serum albumin (g/L)	>35	30–35	<30
B	Serum bilirubin (μmol/L)	<34.2	34.2–51.3	Over >
E	Encephalopathy	Absent	Moderate	Severe
A	Ascites	Absent	Moderate	Tense
N	Nutrition	Good	Moderate	Poor
Pugh's modification replaces nutrition with clotting status:				
	Prothrombin time			
	Seconds prolonged **or**	<4	4 to 6	>6
	% or	>60	40 to 60	<40
	International normalised ratio (INR)	<1.7	1.7 to 2.3	>2.3
	(Score: A = 5–6, B = 7–9, C = 10–15)			

The score can then be used to stratify the severity of disease into three categories. A total score of 5–6 is considered grade A (well-compensated disease); 7–9 is grade B (significant functional compromise); and 10–15 is grade C (decompensated disease). These grades correlate with 1- and 2-year patient survival.

Grade	Points	1-year survival (%)	2-year survival (%)
A: well-compensated disease	5–6	100	85
B: significant functional compromise	7–9	80	60
C: decompensated disease	10–15	45	35

Decompensated liver disease

■ As considered above, liver disease can become 'decompensated' when there is failure of any of the normal functions of the liver.
■ This can present with features that include:
• (hepatic) jaundice
• bleeding/ecchymosis (bruising) – caused by impaired clotting function
• ascites/oedema – caused by decreased protein synthesis
• neurological impairment such as decreased concentration/confusion – caused by hepatic encephalopathy (toxic metabolites passing through the blood-brain barrier).
■ Causes of decompensation include:
• infection (sepsis)
• hypovolaemia (e.g. secondary to a GI bleed) and renal impairment
• alcohol
• drugs
• underlying disease progression/development of hepatocellular carcinoma.

Paracetamol poisoning

■ Levels >150 mg/kg can cause serious (and potentially fatal) toxicity.
■ This threshold is lower in patients with liver impairment and/or an impairment of hepatic metabolism (e.g. chronic alcohol abuse, enzyme-inducing drugs) or starvation.
■ Normal paracetamol metabolism yields N-acetyl-p-benzoquinone imine (NABQI), a toxic metabolite. Although this is normally inactivated and rendered harmless by glutathione, in settings of excess (e.g. overdose), an abundance of NABQI can lead to toxic cellular necrosis.
■ N-acetylcysteine (NAC) is a precursor to glutathione and can therefore help breakdown toxic NABQI. Its protective effect is greatest within the first 12 h of ingestion (ideally 8 h) and it can decrease mortality.
■ The treatment graph below helps define patients that require NAC, based on paracetamol levels.

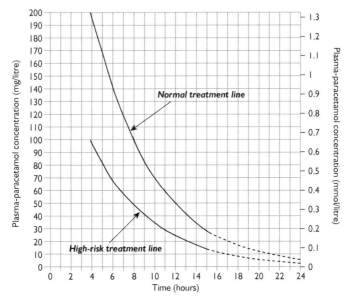

Figure 4.3: Paracetamol overdose treatment curve

Indications for liver transplant

■ While every patient must be assessed for suitability on an individual basis, there are some quantitative investigation-based criteria that can be applied to identify patients suitable for liver transplantation.

■ Broadly speaking, non-liver failure aetiology, specific minimal requirements are:

• immediate need for liver transplantation (i.e. acute liver failure – jaundice and encephalopathy*)

• estimated 1-year post-transplant survival > 90%

• Child-Pugh score > 7 (Child-Pugh class B or C)

• portal hypertensive bleeding or a single episode of spontaneous bacterial peritonitis (irrespective of Child-Pugh score).

*These can be subdivided into hyperacute, acute and subacute.

Disease-specific criteria

NB: These may vary according to centre. The following are based on the Stanford University medical centre criteria (http://med.stanford.edu/shs/txp/livertxp/HTML/selection.adult.html).

Cholestatic liver disease

■ Serum albumin <3.0 g/dL

■ Intractable pruritus

■ Recurrent bacterial cholangitis

Hepatocellular liver disease

- Serum albumin <3.0 g/dL
- Prothrombin time >3 s above control

Both cholestatic and hepatocellular liver disease

- Recurrent or severe hepatic encephalopathy
- Refractory ascites
- Spontaneous bacterial peritonitis (SBP)
- Recurrent portal hypertensive bleeding
- Severe chronic fatigue and weakness
- Progressive malnutrition
- Development of hepatorenal syndrome
- Detection of small, coincidental hepatocellular carcinoma.

Acute fulminant liver failure

Two systems exist.

1 King's College criteria

Paracetamol (acetaminophen) overdose patients

- pH <7.3 **or**
- prothrombin time (as INR) >6.5 **and**
- serum creatinine >3.4 mg/dL

Non-paracetamol (acetaminophen) patients

- prothrombin time (as INR) >6.5 **or**
- any 3 of the following variables:
- 1 age <10 years *or* >40 years
- 2 aetiology: non-A, non-B hepatitis, idiosyncratic drug reaction
- 3 duration of jaundice before encephalopathy >7 days
- 4 prothrombin time (as INR) >3.5
- 5 serum bilirubin >17.6 mg/dL

2 Clichy criteria

Hepatic encephalopathy and:

- Factor V level <20% in patients younger than 30 years of age
- Factor V level <30% in patients 30 year of age or older.

Contraindications to adult liver transplantation

- Extrahepatic malignancy or sepsis.
- Advanced cardiopulmonary disease.
- Active or recent (<6 months) alcohol or substance abuse.

Acute pancreatitis

Causes

The commonest causes in the Western world are alcohol and gallstones. Other causes can be remembered using the mnemonic 'GET SMASHED EPIC'.

Gallstones
EtOH (alcohol)
Trauma

Steroids
Mumps
Autoimmune (e.g. polyarteritis nodosa)
Scorpion venom
Hyperlipidaemia/hypercalcaemia/ hypothermia
ERCP (endoscopic retrograde cholangio-pancreatography)
Drugs (e.g. azathioprine)

Emboli
Pregnancy
Idiopathic
Cancers

Severity stratification

- Scoring systems are used to stratify the severity of the disease. These utilise a number of arterial and venous blood test-based investigative parameters.

■ Although not forming a part of either of the systems below, C-reactive protein (CRP) is another helpful marker; it is perhaps the most useful single marker of disease severity, with serial measurements being useful in monitoring treatment response.

■ Scoring enables serial comparisons to be made and also helps determine management and prognosis.

■ There are two systems in common use.

NB: 1 point awarded for each feature present.

Glasgow criteria
PaO$_2$ (<8 kPa)
Albumin (<32 g/dL)
Neutrophils (WCC >15 × 10^9/L)
Calcium (<2.0 mmol/L)
Raised urea (>16 mmol/L)
Enzymes (LDH 600 IU/L)
AST/ALT (>100 IU/L)
Sugar (glucose >10 mmol/L)

Ranson's criteria
On admission
Sugar (>11.1 mmol/l)
Enzymes (AST > 250 IU/L/ LDH > 350 IU/L)
Age (>55)
Neutrophils (>16 × 10^9/L)

Within 48 h
PaO$_2$ (<8 kPa)
Urea (>1.8 mmol/L)
Sequestered fluid (>6 L)
Haematocrit (>10% fall)
Base excess (>4)
A
Ca^{2+} (<2 mmol/L)
K

Ranson's mortality rate
0–2 : <5% mortality
3–4: 20% mortality
5–6: 40% mortality
7–8: 100% mortality
NB: Other scoring systems also exist, with the Acute Physiology and Chronic Health Evaluation (APACHE)-II system perhaps being the most accurate overall. CT scanning is also a valuable tool in aiding management.

Nutrition

Body Mass Index (BMI)

Used for determining a height-adjusted evaluation of an individual's weight.

$$BMI = \frac{Weight\,(kg)}{Height\,(m^2)}$$

World Health Organization (WHO) defined ranges

Underweight	= <18.4
Normal	= 18.5–24.9
Overweight	= 25.0–29.9
Obese	= 30.0–39.9
Very obese	= >40.0

Vitamin deficiencies

■ Vitamins are organic compounds required through the diet as nutrients, as they cannot be endogenously synthesised in sufficient quantities.

■ Vitamin deficiencies can be either primary (lack of dietary vitamin intake) or secondary (due to an underlying disorder restricting the absorption or use of the vitamin, e.g. excess alcohol intake).

Vitamin	Name of deficiency state	When does deficiency occur?	Clinical features
Water-soluble			
B₁ (thiamine)	Beriberi: 'Dry' (neurologic) Beriberi: 'Wet' (cardiac) Wernicke-Korsakoff syndrome	Refeeding after starvation	Peripheral neuropathy High output heart failure **'NOA'**: **N**ystagmus **O**phthalmoplegia **A**taxia, progressing to anterograde amnesia
B₂ (riboflavin)	–	Rare	Cheilosis, corneal ulcers, glossitis, dermatitis, erythroid hyperplasia
B₃ (niacin)	Pellagra	Poor diet	Dermatitis Dementia Diarrhoea
B₅ (pantothenic acid)		Rare	Dermatitis, adrenal suppression, alopecia
B₆ (pyridoxine)	–	Usually with drugs e.g. isoniazid, cycloserine, penicillamine	Convulsions, anaemia
B₁₂ (cobalamin)	Pernicious anaemia (antibodies against intrinsic factor producing gastric parietal cells)	Achlorhydria	Macrocytic anaemia (+ve Schilling test, raised urinary methylmalonyl)
		Terminal ileal disease or resection	Subacute combined degeneration of the cord: (dorsal columns to lateral columns). Weakness, paraesthesia, loss of proprioception
		Bacterial overgrowth Diphyllobothrium latum	Peripheral neuropathy, Glossitis
		Pancreatic insufficiency	

(Continued)

(Continued)

Vitamin	Name of deficiency state	When does deficiency occur?	Clinical features
Folic acid	–	Pregnancy Poor intake Malabsorption	Macrocytic anaemia (without neurological symptoms), glossitis
Biotin	–	Excess egg white ingestion Total parenteral nutrition	Dermatitis Glossitis Anorexia
C (ascorbic acid)	Scurvy	Infants, elderly and alcoholics. Commonly due to low intake	Purpura/petechia, gum + subperiosteal bleeding, impaired wound healing, perifollicular hyperkeratosis
Fat-soluble			
A (retinol)	–	Poor dietary intake	Night blindness, corneal changes, xerophthalmia, xeroderma and hyperkeratosis
D	–	Inadequate sun exposure Inadequate dietary intake Renal disease	Osteomalacia in adults/rickets in children Hypocalcaemia
E	–	Cholestatic liver disease (especially children)	Erythrocyte fragility, posterior column degeneration, areflexia
K	–	Warfarin (inhibits synthesis) Antibiotics and diarrhoea Neonates (low vit K in breast milk)	Haemorrhage (raised PT). Neonatal bleeds are usually between the 1st and 6th months of life (hence vit K injection given to neonates)

TPN = total parenteral nutrition.

Total parenteral nutrition (TPN)

Although the general rule of thumb is 'enteral is best', several conditions can warrant parenteral feeding (feeding that bypasses the gastrointestinal tract). If gut-based absorption of nutrients is poor (for example, in severe inflammatory bowel diseases) and the patient's body mass index (BMI) and nutritional status have dropped to dangerously low levels, TPN can be initiated via central or peripheral venous access lines.

Absolute indications

■ Enterocutaneous fistulae (high rate of fluid losses); insufficient gut length (e.g. post resection).

Relative indications

■ Moderate to severe malnutrition.
■ Severe inflammatory bowel disease (Crohn's, ulcerative colitis).
■ Acute pancreatitis.
■ Abdominal sepsis.
■ Prolonged ileus.
■ Major trauma/burns.

Feed composition

Peripheral nutrition

■ Hyperosmotic solution (risk of thrombophlebitis, need to change IV cannulas every 1–2 days).
■ Basic composition: 12 g nitrogen and 2000 calories.

Central nutrition

■ Hyperosmolar solution (has a low pH and also irritates to vessel walls).
■ Typically contains (in 2.5 L feed):
• 14 g nitrogen (as L amino acids)
• 250 g glucose
• 500 mL 20% lipid emulsion
• 100 mmol Na^+
• 100 mmol K^+
• 150 mmol Cl^-
• 15 mmol Mg^{2+}
• 13 mmol Ca^{2+}
• 30 mmol PO_4^{2-}
• 0.4 mmol Zn^{2+}
• water and fat-soluble vitamins
• trace elements.

Investigations to monitor TPN

■ TPN requires regular monitoring to prevent the complications associated with over- or under-delivery of the various components of the feed.
■ These complications include electrolyte derangements, deranged liver function tests (LFTs) and deficiency of the various trace elements.
■ Twice-weekly measurements of: Mg^{2+}, Ca^{2+}, PO_4^{2-}, Zn^{2+}, FBC, urea and electrolytes (U&Es), LFTs, nitrogen balance.
■ Blood cultures and removal of lines if sign of sepsis (lines only to be used for feeding).
■ Weight monitoring.

Histological findings in GI disease

Different gastrointestinal pathologies have characteristic histological appearances. The following table describes both macroscopic and microscopic features.

Inflammatory bowel disease

Crohn's disease	■ transmural inflammation
	■ skip lesions (anywhere from mouth to anus)
	■ 'cobblestone' mucosa
	■ ulcers, fissures, granulomata
Ulcerative colitis	■ superficial inflammation
	■ large bowel only
	■ ulcers, crypt abscesses

Liver

Alcoholic hepatitis	▪ fatty deposition (in vacuoles) and extra-lobular fibrosis ▪ Mallory's hyaline bodies (eosinophilic keratin filament inclusions in hepatocytes)
Autoimmune hepatitis	▪ interface hepatitis ▪ portal plasma cell infiltration
Chronic active hepatitis	▪ piecemeal necrosis
Cirrhosis	▪ fibrosis (macro/micronodular) ▪ (chronic) inflammatory cells in fibrous band of portal region ▪ red on Gieson's stain
Non-alcoholic steato hepatitis (NASH)	▪ macrovesicular steatosis (fat accumulation) ▪ lobular inflammation ▪ hepatocyte degeneration (Mallory hyaline – less prominent than in alcoholic hepatitis) ▪ peri-cellular fibrosis → cirrhosis
Viral hepatitis	▪ signs of hepatocellular injury (e.g. Councilman body: eosinophilic globule formed through apoptotic death of a hepatocyte) ▪ hepatocyte inflammation and swelling (inflammatory cells; primarily involving parenchyma, but also the portal areas and inter-connecting 'interface' areas) ▪ evidence of hepatocellular degeneration (spotty necrosis, ballooning, acidophilic bodies) ▪ evidence of hepatocellular regeneration (Kupffer cells; attempt to repair damage) ▪ overall changes are fibrotic and necro-inflammatory (various classification systems exist, e.g. Ishak, METAVIR) ▪ progression: begins as portal expansion → bridging fibrosis between central and portal tracts → cirrhosis

Biliary tract

Cholecystitis (chronic)	■ (chronic) inflammatory cells ■ thickened wall ■ prominent Rokitansky-Aschoff sinuses
Primary biliary cirrhosis	■ granulomas and portal inflammation ■ intralobular bile stasis ■ duct destruction → proliferation ■ portal → peri-portal fibrosis/inflammation ■ later fibrous septa and nodules
Primary sclerosing cholangitis	■ liver histology can resemble chronic active hepatitis ■ periductal fibrosis with inflammation ■ bile duct proliferation ■ ductopaenia

Others

Barrett's (oesophagus)	■ metaplasia (change in type) of epithelium from squamous to columnar (gut-type)
Coeliac disease	■ villous atrophy (small bowel) ■ mucosal inflammation ■ crypt hyperplasia
Haemochromatosis	■ iron excess (blue on Perl's stain)
Wilson's disease	■ signs of chronic active hepatitis ■ Mallory's bodies (as in alcoholic hepatitis) ■ copper deposition

Chapter 5
ENDOCRINOLOGY

Introduction

With a number of established and logical investigative protocols, endocrine disorders often feature prominently in medical examinations. Diabetes mellitus, in particular, is a common condition, the complications of which affect a number of organ systems. This chapter focuses on the conditions more commonly encountered – either in medical examinations or in clinical practice – and attempts to provide a framework for developing an understanding of their pathological basis and diagnosis. As with all investigations, it is especially important in endocrine tests to consider any results in the clinical context.

Topics covered
- Glucose metabolism and diabetes mellitus
- Thyroid disease
- Pituitary hormones
- Adrenal hormones
- Calcium, phosphate and bone diseases
- Multiple endocrine neoplasia (MEN)

Glucose metabolism and diabetes mellitus (DM)

Fasting glucose

Normal range: 3.5–6.0 mmol/L

Low
- Hypoglycaemia

High
- Impaired fasting glucose/tolerance
- Diabetes mellitus (DM)
- Gestational DM (new onset during pregnancy – usually normalises after birth, but does suggest an increased risk of subsequently developing DM)

Oral Glucose Tolerance Test (OGTT)

This test can be used in the diagnosis of DM and to distinguish between the other causes of hyperglycaemia.
- The patient should fast overnight (10 h).
- An initial fasting blood glucose should be taken (baseline).
- This is followed by an oral dose of 75 g glucose in 300 mL water, taken over 5 min.
- A further blood glucose specimen is taken 2 h after the glucose load.

The hands-on guide to data interpretation. By S. Abraham, K. Kulkarni, R. Madhu and D. Provan. Published 2010 by Blackwell Publishing Ltd.

Venous plasma glucose levels (mmol/L)

	Fasting glucose	2 h post oral glucose load (oGTT)
Normal	<6.1	<7.8
Impaired fasting glucose/ glucose tolerance	6.1–6.9	7.8–11.0
Diabetes Mellitus	≥7.0	≥11.1

Diabetes mellitus

Symptoms
■ Polyuria
■ Polydipsia
■ Weight loss
■ Fatigue/malaise
■ Blurred vision
■ May present with diabetic ketoacidosis (DKA)
■ May present with complications of DM (e.g. abscesses, ulcers, etc.)

Diagnosis
■ Symptoms of DM plus:
• single random venous glucose concentration ≥11.1 mmol/L (need 2 × positive tests in asymptomatic patients) **or**
• single fasting venous plasma glucose concentration ≥7.0 mmol/L (need 2 × positive tests in asymptomatic patients) **or**
• plasma glucose concentration ≥11.1 mmol/L, 2 h after 75 g anhydrous glucose (or equivalent) in an OGTT.

Diabetic ketoacidosis (DKA)
■ A life-threatening acute complication of diabetes mellitus, occurring when insulin therapy is absent or becomes inadequate for the current physiological state, usually as a result of intercurrent illness.
■ Although infection is often the trigger, myocardial infarction and other causes can also be implicated, with 50% having no identifiable cause.
■ It may represent the first presentation of diabetes, particularly in children. Usually associated with type-1 DM (patients with type-2 DM are more likely to suffer hyperosmolar non-ketotic coma, or 'HONK', a condition characterised by hyperglycaemia, dehydration and decreased consciousness).
■ Presents as an unwell patient with symptoms/signs including pyrexia, abdominal pain, nausea and vomiting, progressive thirst (dehydration), lassitude/weakness, confusion.

Biochemical features
■ Hyperglycaemia
■ Ketosis
■ Metabolic acidosis

Investigations
■ Urine:
• dipstick reveals marked glycosuria and ketonuria (also send urine for microscopy and culture).
■ Blood:
• plasma glucose: elevated
• full blood count: often a raised WCC (not necessarily indicative of sepsis)
• electrolytes: Na^+ may be high due to dehydration; K^+ may be normal/high due to effect of acidosis (but overall total body K^+ is low)

• urea and creatinine: elevated due to pre-renal renal failure or where renal impairment is the primary cause
• cardiac enzymes (e.g. troponin): may be raised if underlying MI
• CK: raised if rhabdomyolysis or with MI
• amylase: pancreatitis as trigger
• blood cultures: infection as trigger.
■ Arterial blood gas: metabolic acidosis; pCO_2/pO_2 usually normal.
NB: Assay of blood ketones is more sensitive and specific in detecting ketonaemia but is not always available.

Hypoglycaemia

This usually means a venous plasma glucose level of <3.5 mmol/L. Note that the classic symptoms of hypoglycaemia can occur at different levels of glucose.

Causes

■ Excess exogenous insulin or oral hypoglycaemic agents (OHG). This can occur in patients who have taken too much insulin or OHG, who have taken insufficient carbohydrate with their meal or people without diabetes who wish to deliberately self-harm.
■ Endogenous insulin excess (e.g. insulinoma – raised C-peptide and insulin levels).
■ Liver disease (impaired gluconeogenesis).
■ Alcohol.

C-peptide

■ Pro-insulin is released from the pancreas and cleaved to form insulin and C-peptide (amino acids).
■ Low or undetectable levels of C-peptide with normal or high levels of insulin are present in cases of exogenous insulin administration.

HbA1c (glycosylated haemoglobin)

■ Red cell haemoglobin is non-enzymatically glycosylated at a low rate according to the prevailing level of glucose.
■ The percentage of glycosylated haemoglobin provides an accurate estimate of mean glucose levels over the preceding six-weeks, i.e. an estimate of **long-term** glycaemic control.
■ *High* levels therefore indicate *poor* glycaemic control.
■ In patients with abnormal haemoglobin pathologies (e.g. sickle cell), the plasma protein **fructosamine** levels may be used instead to measure glycaemia control over the past few weeks (a shorter timeframe than HbA1c).
■ Fructosamine values do not depend on red cell life span or renal function.

HbA1c values

HbA1c range	Suggests average blood glucose of approx	Explanation
4.0–6.5%	3–8 mmol/L	Normal range (for those without DM)
6.5–7.5%	8–10 mmol/L	Target range (for most patients with DM)
8.0–9.5%	11–14 mmol/L	High
>9.5%	>15 mmol/L	Very high

Abnormally low HbA1c

■ Haemolysis
■ Increased red cell turnover

- Blood loss
- Recent blood (packed red cell) transfusion
- HbS or HbC

Abnormally high HbA1c
- Rare – reported cases with Hb mutations and uraemia, etc.

Complications of DM
- DM is associated with a range of long-term microvascular, macrovascular and neurological complications.
- These include: cardiovascular disease, renal disease, visual loss (retinopathy), erectile dysfunction and neuropathy (peripheral sensory loss and autonomic).
- It is important to screen for these regularly. Some tests include the following.
- Urine dip: the presence of protein can be used to screen for renal disease.
- Blood tests: aside from those monitoring glycaemic control, the higher risk of cardiovascular disease means that cholesterol should be measured. Urea and electrolytes should also be monitored (for renal complications).
- Electrocardiogram (ECG): more relevant in investigating ischaemia/infarcts.
- Fundoscopy/slit lamp examination: to screen for diabetic retinopathy and associated visual loss. *NB:* the gold standard investigation is retinal photography using a slit lamp.

Thyroid disease

- T4 and T3 are produced by the thyroid gland and are stimulated by TSH from the anterior pituitary (which in itself is stimulated by thyrotrophin-releasing hormone (TRH) from the hypothalamus). The process is regulated by negative feedback of T4 and T3 on the pituitary gland.
- While most plasma T4 and T3 is bound to thyroxine-binding globulin (TBG), it is the free component of these hormones that is active.
- A number of primary endocrine abnormalities can affect the thyroid gland. Secondary abnormalities (affecting TRH/TSH) are considerably rarer.

Hypothalamic-pituitary axis

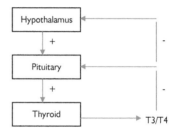

Figure 5.1: Hypothalamic-pituitary axis; note how T3 and T4 provide negative feedback

Investigations

- Blood tests: total/free T4, T3 and TSH. TRH-test (rarely performed).
- Immunology: thyroid antibodies, thyroid stimulating immunoglobulin.
- Radioisotope studies: thyroid uptake studies.
- Ultrasound.
- Fine needle aspiration (FNA – for cytology, or cellular architecture) or histology (of gross tissue architecture, after surgical resection – hemi/subtotalthyroidectomy).

Thyroid function tests

	TSH	**T3**	**T4**
Normal range (free)	0.4–5 mU/L	5–10 pmol/L	10–22 pmol/L
Normal range (total)	0.4–5 mU/L	1.07–3.18 nmol/L	58–174 nmol/L
Euthyroid	N	N	N
Primary hypothyroidism	H	L	L
Secondary hypothyroidism	L/N	L	L
Primary hyperthyroidism (thyrotoxicosis)	L	H	H
Secondary hyperthyroidism (e.g. tumour) – rare	N/H	H	H
Sick euthyroid syndrome (e.g. during acute illness)	L/N	L	L
T3 thyrotoxicosis	L	H	N

NB: Most laboratories now offer free hormone assays for T3 and T4 (see Chapter 1). Please note that normal ranges may vary between laboratories and healthy individuals.

H = high, L = low, N = normal.

Hyperthyroidism: primary causes

- Graves' disease
- Thyroid nodules ('hyper-functioning' – toxic adenoma, toxic multi-nodular goitre, follicular carcinoma – although patients can often be euthyroid)
- Thyroiditis (e.g. postpartum, sub-acute, etc.)
- Iodine excess (dietary; drugs, e.g. amiodarone)
- Excess thyroxine replacement
- Subacute (De Quervain's)

Eye signs of Graves' disease
- Grade 0 = no signs or symptoms
- Grade 1 = only signs, no symptoms
- Grade 2 = soft tissue involvement
- Grade 3 = proptosis
- Grade 4 = extraocular muscle involvement
- Grade 5 = corneal involvement
- Grade 6 = sight loss with optic involvement

Hypothyroidism: causes

Primary
- Hashimoto's thyroiditis (autoimmune)
- Post-thyroidectomy
- Post-radio-iodine thyroid treatment
- External beam radiation (e.g. for treatment of lymphomas)
- Drugs (e.g. excess anti-thyroid drugs, amiodarone)
- Iodine deficiency

Secondary
- Pituitary/hypothalamic pathology (e.g. post surgery)

Thyroid antibodies

Thyroid peroxidase antibody	Hashimoto's thyroiditis, Graves' disease
Thyroglobulin	Thyroid malignancy, Hashimoto's thyroiditis
Thyroid stimulating hormone receptor antibody	Graves' disease

Pituitary hormones

■ There are six hormones produced by the anterior pituitary and two produced by the posterior part of the gland.
■ Problems with the pituitary gland can therefore have a range of different presentations.

Anterior pituitary (adenohypophysis) – 'FLAT PIG'

FSH (follicle-stimulating hormone)
LH (luteinising hormone)
ACTH
TSH

Prolactin
(I)
Growth hormone (GH)

Posterior pituitary (neurohypophysis) – 'OA'

Oxytocin
ADH (anti-diuretic hormone or vasopressin)
NB: For more detail on the reproductive hormones, please see Chapter 10.

Pituitary function tests

■ A number of tests, designed to stimulate the hypothalamo-pituitary axis, can provide indication of pituitary function.
■ These include TRH (thyrotrophin-releasing hormone) test, luteinising hormone releasing hormone (LHRH) (in pre-menopausal women) and LH/FSH tests (in post-menopausal women), insulin stress test and water deprivation test.
■ Some of these will be considered in more detail in this section.

Growth hormone (GH): acromegaly

■ This is a condition associated with excess growth hormone (GH).
■ It is usually secondary to a pituitary tumour.
Features include:
■ *Symptoms:* increase in sizes (e.g. of shoes and rings), sweating, headache, local tumour mass effects (focal neurology).
■ *Signs:* characteristic 'enlargement' (macroglossia, spade-like hands, prognathism, prominent supraorbital ridge), heart failure, hypopituitarism, focal neurology.

Investigation
■ Gold standard for diagnosis: oral glucose tolerance test (OGTT): as used in investigating diabetes mellitus, normal = growth hormone levels <2 mU/L (some centres use <1 mU/L), acromegaly = failure to suppress, or even a paradoxical rise.
■ Insulin-like grown factor (IGF-1): marker of average GH levels (over the past day) – high levels indicate excess GH secretion.

■ Isolated GH measurements (not diagnostic or reliable, as levels vary during the day).

■ Imaging of pituitary fossa (usually by MRI).

■ Others: compare appearance with old photos (to assist diagnosis), electrocardiogram (ECG) or cardiac echo scan (to look for complications).

Normal range: <1 mU/L (basal, fasting and between pulses), >40 mU/L (after hypoglycaemia, many centres accept values >20 mU/L)

Prolactin

■ This is one of the hormones responsible for normal milk secretion from the breast.

■ High levels can cause galactorrhoea.

■ Prolactin is under indirect positive feedback control by dopamine (dopamine from the hypothalamus has an inhibitory effect on the synthesis and secretion of prolactin).

Increased (directly elevated prolactin)

■ Pregnancy and breast-feeding
■ Oestrogens
■ Polycystic ovary syndrome
■ Tumours (prolactinoma – can be associated with very high levels, e.g. >5000 mIU/L). These can be micro (<10 mm) or macro (>10 mm)
■ Hypothyroidism
■ Post-seizure

Increased (interruption of dopaminergic inhibitory tone)

■ Drugs (e.g. phenothiazines, such as haloperidol, or anti-emetics, such as metoclopramide)
■ Damage to pituitary stalk (e.g. pressure from a pituitary tumour)
■ Damage to hypothalamus

Decreased

■ Dopamine agonist (e.g. bromocriptine)

Investigation

■ Basal plasma prolactin (usually measured during the daytime).
■ Imaging (CT/MRI) of the gland if levels are elevated (e.g. >1000 mIU/L) to exclude underlying pathology.

Normal range: 65–490 mIU/L (females), 55–340 mIU/L (males)

Antidiuretic hormone (ADH)

■ ADH acts on the distal tubule of the kidneys to increase water resorption (conserve water).

Diabetes insipidus (DI)

■ This is a condition associated with either abnormal ADH secretion from the posterior pituitary (central) or an abnormal renal response to ADH (nephrogenic).
■ Symptoms/signs therefore include polyuria, polydipsia and dilute urine.
■ The main differential diagnosis is psychogenic polydipsia (excess water drinking).

Water deprivation test

- Used to identify the cause of polydipsia (excessive thirst) and/or polyuria (excessive diuresis).
- Major metabolic causes should be excluded first (e.g. hyperglycaemia, hypercalcaemia, hypokalaemia, chronic renal failure).

Protocol

- The patient is deprived of water (from the night before if polyuria is not excessive).

- Hourly urine and plasma osmolarity are measured until 3% of the body weight is lost (or until the serum sodium rises/urine becomes concentrated).
- The patient is then given an injection of DDAVP (a synthetic analogue of ADH).

	Initial plasma osmolality	Final plasma osmolality	Final urine osmolality mOsm/kg	Urine osmolality post DDAVP mOsm/kg
Normal	Normal	Normal	>600	>600
Cranial DI	High	Normal	<300	>600
Nephrogenic DI	High	High	<300	<300
Primary polydipsia	Low	Relatively low	300–400	400
Partial cranial DI	High	Relatively high	300–400	400–600

Cranial DI = problem with central release of ADH.
Nephrogenic DI = lack of renal response to ADH.

Syndrome of inappropriate ADH secretion (SIADH)

This is a cause of hyponatraemia (low sodium, Na^+).

Diagnostic criteria

- Euvolaemia
- Normal endocrine function (euthyroid, no renal or adrenal disease)
- Hyponatraemia
- Low serum osmolality
- Urine osmolality > serum osmolality (concentrated urine, urine osmolality usually > 500 mosmol/kg, serum osmolality <260 mosmol/kg)
- Urinary sodium >20 mmol/L

Causes

- Drugs:
  - carbamazepine
  - anti-psychotics.
- Intracranial:
  - tumours
  - infections
  - trauma (head injury).
- Thoracic:
  - tumours (e.g. lung tumours)
  - infections.

Adrenal hormones

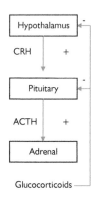

Adrenal cortex
'Deeper is sweeter':
- Zona **G**lomerulosa: mineralocorticoids
- Zona **F**asciculata: glucocorticoids
- Zona **R**eticularis: sex steroids

Adrenal medulla
- Epinephrine
- Norepinephrine

Figure 5.2: Adrenal hormone feedback loop

Cortisol

■ Cortisol is a corticosteroid hormone produced by the adrenal cortex.
■ Cushing's syndrome is caused by an excess of glucocorticoids.

Hypercortisolism (Cushing's syndrome)
Raised cortisol (non-ACTH dependent)
■ Iatrogenic (steroid drugs – common)
■ Adrenal adenoma/carcinoma

Raised cortisol (ACTH dependent)
■ Pituitary tumour (Cushing's disease)
■ Ectopic ACTH production (e.g. small cell lung cancer)
■ Iatrogenic (exogenous ACTH administration, e.g. Synacthen test; otherwise uncommon)

Investigation
■ 24-hour urinary free cortisol
■ Serum cortisol/ACTH levels
■ Dexamethasone suppression tests (overnight, low-dose, high-dose)

> *Normal range:* 09.00h: 200–700 nmol/L; 22.00h: 50–200 nmol/L (normal circadian variation, with cortisol undetectable at midnight)

Diagnosis of Cushing's syndrome
■ It is not possible to diagnose Cushing's syndrome with a single test.
■ Most centres therefore combine the dexamethasone suppression test with an assessment of circadian rhythm +/– a measure of urinary free cortisol estimation.

Dexamethasone suppression test (overnight)

■ This test is used in the investigation of Cushing's disease.

■ Dexamethasone (a steroid) should suppress cortisol levels, by a negative feedback effect.

Overnight test

■ The patient is given a 1 mg tablet of dexamethasone between 22.00 h and 24.00 h.

■ A serum cortisol level is then taken at 09.00 h.

Low-dose test

■ Starting at 09.00h, the patient is given eight doses of 0.5 mg dexamethasone at 6-hourly intervals.

■ Cortisol levels are measured 48 h later.

Both tests: raised cortisol (>50 nmol/L) is suggestive of Cushing's syndrome.

NB: The sensitivity and specificity of the tests is not 100%. False positives can be due to a number of reasons, including excess alcohol intake, obesity and depressive illness.

Hypocortisolism

Reduced cortisol (Addison's disease – primary adrenocortical insufficiency)

■ Autoimmune (80%) – associated with other conditions, e.g. Graves' disease, DM, pernicious anaemia)

■ Infective (e.g. tuberculosis, HIV, cytomegalovirus (CMV))

■ Malignancy (metastasis, lymphoma)

■ Post-infective haemorrhage (Waterhouse-Friederichsen's syndrome – post meningococcal infection)

■ Systemic lupus erythematosus (SLE)

■ Anti-phospholipid syndrome

Short synacthen (synthetic ACTH) test

This is a screening test for cortisol reserves, used to investigate potential Addison's disease (primary adrenocortical insufficiency). A good response to ACTH suggests that there is no primary adrenal disease.

■ A serum cortisol sample is taken at 0 minutes.

■ This is followed by 250 µg Synacthen between 08.00 and 10.00 h.

■ Further serum cortisol specimens are taken at 30 and 60 min after the Synacthen administration.

Increased cortisol >550 nmol/L at 30/60 min = adequate adrenal reserve.

Insulin tolerance test

Less commonly used. In normal individuals, hypoglycaemia (<2.2 mmol/L) induces a normal stress response. This is rising cortisol (>550 nmol/L) and growth hormone levels (>40 mU/L, though most centres accept values >20 mU/L). However, this is more often used to assess ACTH reserve rather than the cortisol reserve.

Indications

■ Cortisol > 100 nmol/L (i.e. not frankly low)

■ Normal thyroid function and no cardiovascular disease

■ No history of epilepsy/seizure activity/blackouts

Congenital adrenal hyperplasias

These are conditions associated with deficiencies in one of a number of enzymes involved in the synthesis of aldosterone, cortisol, testosterone or oestradiol. [1], [2] and [3] refer to the labelled arrows in Figure 5.3.

■ [2] missing = 21-beta-hydroxylase deficiency:

• commonest

• decreased cortisol and mineralocorticoids = low BP & Na$^+$, high K$^+$ & rennin → salt and volume depletion and 'salt wasting crises'

• increased sex hormones = masculinisation (females are 'pseudohermaphrodites').

■ [1] missing = 17-alpha-hydroxylase deficiency:

• decreased sex hormones and cortisol = low K$^+$

• raised mineralocorticoids = high BP

• phenotypic females, but no sexual maturation.

■ [3] missing = 11-beta-hydroxylase deficiency:

• low cortisol and aldosterone

• high sex hormones = masculinisation

• but – high BP (as 11-deoxycorticosterone is a weak mineralocorticoid).

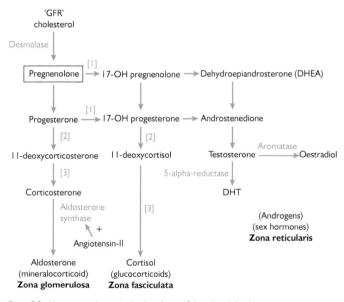

Figure 5.3: Hormone production in the three layers of the adrenal gland

Phaeochromocytoma

■ These are rare adrenal medullary tumours associated with excess production and release of catecholamines.

■ The classic 'rule of 10s' (10% malignant, 10% familial, 10% extra-adrenal,

10% multiple, i.e. bilateral) has been shown to be not strictly true (for example, >10% are known to have a genetic basis and >40% have some malignant association).

■ Familial tumours are associated with multiple endocrine neoplasia (MEN) 2a and b, Von-Hippel Lindau syndrome, type I neurofibromatosis and mutations in the succinate dehydrogenase gene family.

Investigation
Diagnosis
24-hour urine for:

■ first choice: catecholamines (norepinephrine/epinephrine) and their metabolites (metanephrines). However, it is important to remember that these tests are still not available everywhere
■ less commonly used: vanillylmandelic acid (VMA).

Site

■ MIBG (meta-iodo-benzyl-guanidine) scan (to localise tumour).

Hyperaldosteronism

Primary hyperaldosteronism (Conn's syndrome)
Causes

■ Unilateral adrenocortical adenoma (Conn's syndrome) = >50%
■ Bilateral adrenocortical hyperplasia
■ Adrenal carcinoma

Investigations

■ Low K⁺ (20% are normokalaemic)
■ BP raised
■ Raised aldosterone
■ Low rennin

Secondary hyperaldosteronism
Due to a high renin level

Causes

■ Renal artery stenosis
■ Malignant/accelerated hypertension
■ Diuretics
■ Congestive cardiac failure
■ Hepatic failure

Additional investigations

■ Renal Doppler ultrasound/angiography
■ Cardiac echosonography

Calcium, phosphate and bone

Homeostasis of calcium (Ca^{2+}) & phosphate (PO_4^-) involves:

■ the bones, the kidneys and the gut
■ two hormones: parathyroid hormone (PTH) and alkaline phosphatase (ALP)
■ vitamin D.

Calcium

> *Normal range:* 2.12–2.65 mmol/L

Corrected calcium
Calcium in plasma is bound to albumin (protein). It is the unbound component (metabolically active) that is measured. In states of low albumin, this can therefore lead to misleading results. For this reason, 'corrected' calcium is often calculated to compensate for this:

$$Corrected\ Ca^{2+}\ [in\ mmol/L] = measured\ serum\ Ca^{2+}\ [in\ mmol/L] + (0.02 \times (40 - albumin\ [in\ g/L]))$$

Low – causes

■ Vitamin D deficiency
■ Parathyroid disease (e.g. hypoparathyroidism)
■ Surgery (damage to parathyroid glands during neck surgery)
■ Acute rhabdomyolysis

High – causes
Common
- Malignancy (bone metastases, myeloma)
- Primary hyperparathyroidism

Rare
- Thyrotoxicosis
- Sarcoidosis
- Addison's disease
- Vitamin D intoxication
- Familial (benign) hypocalciuric hypercalcaemia

Regulation
If calcium is low, then PTH rises. This results in the following.
- Increased resorption of Ca^{2+} from bone.
- Increased renal reabsorption of Ca^{2+}.
- Increased renal PO_4^- excretion (**P**hosphate **T**rashing **H**ormone).
- (Indirectly) increased Ca^{2+} reabsorption from gut (via vitamin D).

Phosphate

> *Normal range:* 0.8–1.6 mmol/L

Low – causes
- Osteomalacia and rickets
- Drugs: diuretics, antacids, long-term steroid use
- Severely malnourished patient or refeeding syndrome
- Pancreatitis
- Diabetic ketoacidosis (DKA)
- Electrolyte disturbance (e.g. hypokalaemia, or associated with hypercalcaemia of hyperparathyroidism)

High – causes
- Spurious (haemolysis, post-prandial, sample not kept cool)
- Decreased excretion (low glomerular filtration rate, hypoparathyroidism)
- Increased absorption (high vitamin D, high intake)
- Trans-cellular shift (tumour lysis syndrome, soft tissue trauma)
- Dehydration and hypovolaemia

Bone diseases

	Calcium	Phosphate	Alkaline phosphatase
Normal ranges	2.2–2.6 mmol/L	0.8–1.4 mmol/L	45–105 U/L
Osteoporosis	N	N	N
Osteomalacia	L	L	H
Paget's disease	N	N	H
Myeloma	H	H, N	N
Bone metastasis	H	H, N	H
Primary hyperparathyroidism	H	L, N	N, H
Secondary hyperparathyroidism	N, L	H	N, H
Tertiary hyperparathyroidism	H	L	N
Hypoparathyroidism	L	H	N

Key: H = high; L = low; N = normal.

Definitions

Primary hyperparathyroidism: hyperfunction of the parathyroid glands. This can be due to oversecretion of PTH due to adenoma (most common), hyperplasia (usually associated with multiple endocrine neoplasia, MEN) or carcinoma of the parathyroid glands (very rare).

Secondary hyperparathyroidism: parathyroid gland reaction to hypocalcaemia caused by something other than a parathyroid pathology, e.g. chronic renal failure.

Tertiary hyperparathyroidism: excessive secretion of PTH after a long period of secondary hyperparathyroidism (results in hypercalcaemia), e.g. prolonged periods of chronic renal failure.

Multiple endocrine neoplasia (MEN)

■ These are rare syndromes involving the development of either multiple endocrine gland tumours or hyperplasia.
■ Almost all MEN syndromes have a genetic basis.
There are three main types of MEN.

■ MEN 1 (Wermer's syndrome):
• 'Ps': parathyroid (usually adenomas), pancreatic (>50% gastrinomas) or pituitary glands (usually produce prolactin or GH).
■ MEN 2a (Sipple's syndrome):
• medullary carcinoma of thyroid (almost all patients)
• phaeochromocytoma (about 50% patients)
• parathyroid hyperplasia (some patients) – hyperparathyroidism.
■ MEN 2b:
• medullary carcinoma of thyroid
• phaeochromocytoma
• neuromas (especially around mucous membranes, e.g. lips, tongue and mouth, as well as in the gastrointestinal tract and cutaneous).

Investigation

■ Diagnosis of each individual tumour/organ hyperplasia is detected by appropriate investigation of symptoms (e.g. hormone assays, imaging, etc.).
■ Genetic screening is important due to inherited nature of condition – involves genetic testing for individual gene mutations.

Chapter 6
RENAL

Introduction

This chapter considers the interpretation of data relating to investigations of the urinary tract. It will consider some of the commonly used tools such as blood tests and urine dipstick, and will also provide an overview of the main imaging modalities that can be used to visualise the urinary tract. Finally, we will discuss some of the important renal pathologies.

Topics covered
- Urinary tract imaging
- Urinalysis
- Urine microscopy
- Urine cytology
- Renal biopsy
- Urea, creatinine and electrolytes
- Prostate specific antigen (PSA)
- Calculi
- Polycystic kidney disease (PKD)
- Nephrotic syndrome
- Nephritic syndrome (glomerulonephritis)
- Acute versus chronic renal failure
- Anion gap

Urinary tract imaging

- The urinary tract includes the kidneys, ureters, bladder, prostate (in men) and the urethra.
- The appropriate choice of investigation to visualise the urinary tract depends on the clinical history and examination findings.
- There are a number of indications for imaging the urinary tract. While detailed discussion of these is beyond the scope of this chapter, some indications include:
- lower urinary tract symptoms (e.g. frequency, urgency, dysuria, poor stream, incontinence, etc.)
- haematuria
- oliguria/anuria (and other symptoms/signs of acute/chronic renal failure)
- abdominal masses/pain
- uncontrolled hypertension.

Available modalities include the following.

X-ray
- Abdominal 'KUB' (kidney, ureter, bladder) films.
- Can visualise calculi (80–90% are radio-opaque), and other pathologies causing calcification (e.g. malignancy, tuberculosis).

The hands-on guide to data interpretation. By S. Abraham, K. Kulkarni, R. Madhu and D. Provan. Published 2010 by Blackwell Publishing Ltd.

Intravenous urogram/pyelogram (IVU/IVP) series

■ This involves a series of abdominal X-ray films taken before and at several intervals after injection of an IV contrast agent.

■ It allows visualisation of the anatomy of the pelvi-calyceal and collecting systems, as well as the ureters and bladder. Its primary role is therefore in the investigation of urinary tract obstruction.

■ To obtain a retrograde pyelogram, contrast is injected via a catheter.

■ A percutaneous nephrostomy allows contrast to be injected directly into the kidneys. This procedure is also therapeutic as it also allows drainage of urine (e.g. if there is an outflow obstruction).

■ Note that IVU is increasingly being replaced by the computed tomography urogram (CTU) (see below).

Ultrasound (trans-abdominal)

■ This safe and non-invasive technique is often used for visualisation of renal size (small in chronic failure, large with masses, e.g. in polycystic kidney disease, unilateral kidney compensatory functional hypertrophy).

■ It is commonly used to detect hydronephrosis and fluid collections.

■ Ultrasound is also useful for measuring bladder residual volume.

■ Note that ultrasound is not as sensitive/specific as other modalities such as CT for imaging ureteral obstruction.

Transrectal ultrasound (TRUS)

■ Usually used to detect irregularities of the prostate by allowing the transducer to come directly into contact with it. Also used to aid prostate biopsies.

Computed tomography (CT) and CT urogram (CTU)

■ Very sensitive for detection of stones and determining the characteristics of masses (e.g. renal tumours).

■ Like MRI, CT can be used with a radio-opaque contrast agent to enhance the imaging of masses and to evaluate vascular pathology.

■ CT urogram (CTU) has now taken over from IVU/P (intravenous urogram/ pyelogram) as the investigation of choice for calculi.

■ The advantages of CTU (performed without contrast) are increased sensitivity for stone detection, increased speed, avoidance of potential adverse reactions to contrast, less dependence on renal function and decreased radiation exposure.

Magnetic resonance imaging (MRI)

■ Better visualisation of soft tissue masses. Can be used for investigating renal artery stenosis (although the gold standard remains angiography).

■ MR angiography (MRA) is now used routinely instead of invasive angiography for imaging of the renal artery. Note that if performed with contrast (e.g. gadolinium), there is a potential risk of adverse reactions to the contrast, notably in pregnancy or in patients with impaired renal failure (i.e. reduced glomerular filtration rate, GFR).

Renal arteriography (angiography)

■ This has diagnostic uses (such as detection of renal artery stenosis) as well as a therapeutic role (stenting, angioplasty, embolisation of bleeding points).

■ As an invasive procedure, complications include vascular/adjacent organ damage and bleeding, as well as possible reaction to the contrast agent.

■ Its role in diagnosis of renal artery pathology is has now been largely superseded by the more sensitive and less invasive MRA (see *above*).

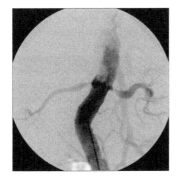

Figure 6.1: Renal angiogram

Micturating cysturethrogram (MCUG)

■ Less commonly used in adults.

■ A catheter is used to place contrast into the bladder and X-rays are taken as the patient voids.

■ It is sometimes used to visualise vesico-ureteric reflux (a cause of recurrent infections), or to see if there is an abnormality of the urinary tract causing persistent infection in children.

$^{99}Tc^m$Diethylene triamine penta-acetic acid (DTPA), mercapto acetyl tri glycine (Mag-3) and dimercaptosuccinic acid (DMSA) cortical scintigraphy

■ These investigations have slightly different roles in the investigation of renal function.

■ They are often used in children, e.g. to assess renal function a few months after urinary tract infection (UTI).

■ DMSA: this 'static' 99-technetium (^{99}Tc)-based investigation can be used to assess anatomical information about the kidneys, e.g. to detect renal scarring (e.g. after pyelonephritis). In children it is often used during/after UTI to assess for progression of scarring/hypertrophy (i.e. abnormal size of kidney), as well as to detect anatomical abnormalities such as duplex kidney.

■ DTPA/Mag-3: this 'dynamic' renal scan can be used to assess aspects of renal function such as renal blood flow (e.g. assessment of the renal artery pre-transplant) and filtration. After the radioactive agent is administered IV, a gamma camera is used to track its passage through the renal vasculature and the kidney itself.

■ The investigations are usually performed at specialist centres.

See Chapter 15 for further details.

Urethroscopy, cystocopy and ureteroscopy

■ These endoscopic procedures can be used to directly visualise the urethera, bladder and ureter respectively.

■ They employ similar (albeit smaller) flexible telescopic cameras to other types of endoscopy, such as gastrointestinal endoscopy.

■ Some indications include the investigation of recurrent UTI or haematuria, and extraction of calculi.

See Chapter 15 for more details about the specifics of each of these.

Urinalysis

■ Urine dipstick is one of the most useful basic investigations for helping to diagnose urinary tract pathology.

■ It is often used in cases of suspected UTI, and can also be useful in screening for conditions such as diabetes and hypertension, with end organ damage being reflected through the presence of glucose and protein respectively.

■ Samples collected should be of 'midstream' urine (i.e. after having already passed a small amount of urine).

■ There are usually 10 components to a dipstick reading (normal reading in brackets).

1 Blood (negative)

■ Detects free haemoglobin and myoglobin, as well as red blood cells (hence false positives).

■ Causes: infection, malignancy, stones, trauma (e.g. catheterisation), hydronephrosis, renal disease (polycystic, parenchymal), inflammation (interstitial cystitis), coagulopathies, antiplatelet/anticoagulant drugs (but do not attribute haematuria solely to drugs without investigating other causes first).

■ False positives: certain foods (beetroot), drugs (rifampicin, phenidone, phenolphthalein), metabolic disorders (porphyria).

2 Protein (negative)

■ Aside from trace amounts of (normal) Tamm-Horsfall proteins, most is reabsorbed by the kidneys. This is usually clinically undetectable.

■ Uses a pH dye indicator (sensitive for albumin, less so for Bence Jones proteins, etc.).

■ Interpret with the specific gravity. Trace proteinuria with a low specific gravity = significant loss. However, this is not the case with high specific gravity.

■ Elevated with UTI, fever, exercise, pregnancy, diabetes mellitus, glomerulonephritis, hypertension.

■ Proteinuria = >150 mg/day (suggestive of diabetes mellitus, hypertension, lupus, glomerulonephritis).

■ Macroalbuminuria = >300 mg/day. Note that microalbuminuria (30–300 mg/day) is not routinely detected with dipsticks and that urine includes proteins other than albumin.

3 Glucose (negative)

■ Normally freely filtered and fully reabsorbed.

■ Positive in low renal threshold states (e.g. chronic renal failure), diabetes mellitus, pregnancy, sepsis, renal tubular damage.

4 Ketones (negative)

■ Acetone, acetoacetic acid, beta-hydroxybutyric acid.

■ Elevated in starvation, diabetic ketoacidosis, insulinoma, high-fat and low-carbohydrate diets, glycogen storage diseases.

5 Leucocytes (negative)

■ Elevated in genitourinary tract infections renal calculi, analgesic nephropathy.

■ False negatives when patients have already commenced antibiotic therapy.

6 Nitrites (negative)

■ Elevated with certain bacterial infections (especially Gram-negative rods), high-protein meals.

■ Ideally requires urine to have been held in the bladder for >4 h (hence a morning sample is useful).

■ Low-sensitivity test (lots of false negatives).

7 Bilirubin (negative)

■ Conjugated bilirubin found in obstructive (post-hepatic) jaundice.

8 Urobilinogen (positive)

■ Formed by intestinal breakdown of conjugated bilirubin, small amounts of which are reabsorbed and excreted in urine.

■ Positive tests indicate a normal entero-hepatic circulation.

■ Elevated levels in pre-hepatic jaundice (e.g. haemolysis) or intestinal dysfunction.

9 Specific gravity (1.002–1.035)

■ Measure of renal concentrating ability.

■ Ratio of urine weight:weight of equivalent volume of water.

10 pH (4.4–5.3)

■ Normal range varies with several factors, including diet.

■ Can get false positives with glycosuria.

NB: For more details about the role of urinalysis in the investigation of infection, please see Chapter 13.

Urine microscopy

■ This should also be performed on a mid-stream specimen of urine, obtained by a 'clean'-catch technique. This involves first cleaning the genital area, then retracting the foreskin (men) or parting the labia (women) before passing urine. Alternatively, a specimen taken through a supra-pubic catheter can be used.

■ A common use for microscopy can be in female patients with recurrent UTI. Remember that all men and children with suspected UTI should be investigated. Another use is in the investigation of suspected renal disease.

The components include the following.

Leucocytes

■ Normal = <10 white blood cells per microlitre or high power field (HPF) in an unspun urine specimen.

■ Elevated in: infections (cystitis, urethritis, prostatitis, pyelonephritis, glomerulonephritis, interstitial nephritis, tuberculosis), renal calculi, analgesia nephropathy.

Red cells

■ Microscopic: >3 erythrocytes/high power field in sediment analysis.

■ Macroscopic: visible with <0.5 mL blood/500 mL urine.

Casts

Cylindrical bodies formed in the lumen of the distal tubule.

■ Hyaline:

• normal (clear and colourless)

• formed by the solidification of Tamm-Horsfall proteins

• may be elevated after exercise, fever or use of loop diuretics.

■ Cellular:

• leucocyte – renal infection or inflammation (pyelonephritis)

• epithelial – tubular damage

• red blood cell – renal infection or inflammation (glomerulonephritis)

• bacterial – renal bacterial infection.

■ Granular:

• formed by the breakdown of cellular casts or from the inclusion of aggregates of plasma proteins, fibrinogen or immune complexes

• often associated with glomerulonephritis, diabetic nephropathy, amyloidosis, interstitial nephritis.

■ Waxy:

• from the final degradation of cellular or granular casts

• seen in chronic renal failure or stasis.

■ Others:
• Fatty (associated with proteinuria), pigment, crystal (urate, calcium oxalate, cysteine).

Urine cytology

■ This involves microscopic examination of cells present in the urine.

■ Its primary investigative use is in the diagnosis/follow-up of malignancy (e.g. bladder cancer), particularly in symptomatic patients. It can also play a role in the screening of malignancy in those at high risk (e.g. exposure to certain industrial chemicals, smokers, schistosomiasis).

■ For example, in the detection of bladder cancers, it should be used after consideration of the clinical context (history and examination) and in conjunction with cystoscopy +/– biopsy. In this instance, a patient may present with haematuria, warranting further investigation.

■ Other investigative uses include inflammatory disorders (including certain infections) and calculi or crystal disease.

■ Mid-morning/random urine samples are preferable for cytological examination.

Renal biopsy

■ This involves taking a specimen of renal tissue, usually using a percutaneous (needle-based) technique.

■ Biopsy is usually image guided (e.g. with ultrasound or CT), with open or 'blind' biopsy being very uncommon nowadays. Pre-biopsy imaging is usually preformed with ultrasound in order to confirm the presence of two non-obstructed kidneys.

■ Uses include:
• the investigation of certain cases of acute renal failure (e.g. to exclude acute tubular necrosis)
• post-transplant (e.g. to determine cause of failure/rejection)
• determining the cause of glomerular or interstitial disease (e.g. glomerulonephritis and related disorders, proteinuria, haematuria suspected to be caused by upper tract pathology).

■ Contraindications include: patients with chronic renal failure and subsequently shrunken kidneys, acute pyelonephritis, uncontrolled hypertension or bleeding diathesis. Presence of only a single kidney is a relative contraindication.

Urea, creatinine and electrolytes

Urea

■ Urea is another waste product formed by the breakdown of nitrogenous compounds (primarily from the deamination of amino acids to urea and ammonia).

■ It is affected by protein and water intake.

■ In the nephrons, urea plays an important role in establishing the countercurrent system (for reabsorption of water and other electrolytes).

■ Particularly in the elderly, a common cause for an isolated urea rise is dehydration.

■ When investigating urea rises, it can be helpful to consider the relative rise of urea with respect to any risk in creatinine.

Normal range: 3–7 mmol/L

Increased urea (proportionally more than creatinine)
- Dehydration
- Infection
- Pre-renal failure/acute-on-chronic renal failure
- Gastrointestinal haemorrhage
- Drugs (e.g. steroids/tetracycline)
- Surgery
- High protein diet

Decreased urea (less commonly encountered)
- Liver disease (e.g. secondary to alcohol)
- Starvation/anabolic state
- Raised anti-diuretic hormone (ADH)
- Pregnancy

Creatinine

- Creatinine is a waste product formed by the natural breakdown of muscle cells; those with higher muscle mass will have a higher baseline creatinine.
- It accumulates in the blood with impaired renal function (e.g. acute/chronic renal failure).
- In clinical use, it is used in conjunction with the 'urea and electrolytes' ('U&E') blood test.
- As there are many potential causes of a raised creatinine, it can be helpful to consider it in conjunction with any elevation of urea: see if the urea and creatinine have increased proportionally. Disproportionate increases of one over the other can yield clues as to the aetiology of the pathology.

Normal range: 70–150 mmol/L (dependent on muscle bulk)

Increased creatinine (proportional rise with urea)
- Renal failure
- Increased catabolism (sepsis, trauma, surgery)
- Pyelonephritis
- Decreased tubular secretion (e.g. K^+ sparing diuretics)

Increased creatinine (proportionally greater rise than urea)
- Drugs (e.g. trimethoprim, co-trimoxazole)
- Hepatic failure
- Rhabdomyolysis

Decreased creatinine
- Small muscle mass
- Pregnancy
- Raised ADH

Electrolytes

Hyponatraemia – low sodium (Na^+)
Approach to investigation

- Hyponatraemia is a common finding on a blood test. However, there are many causes, and it is therefore particularly important to consider the clinical context.
- It can also be helpful to look at previous blood test results: has there been a trend of decreasing sodium levels or is this an isolated reading that should be repeated to exclude an erroneous reading?
- The next step in the investigation of hyponatraemia is to consider the patient's volume status: are they euvolaemic (normal fluid balance), hypervolaemic (fluid over-loaded) or hypovolaemic (dehydrated)?
- The following flow chart can help narrow down the potential causes.

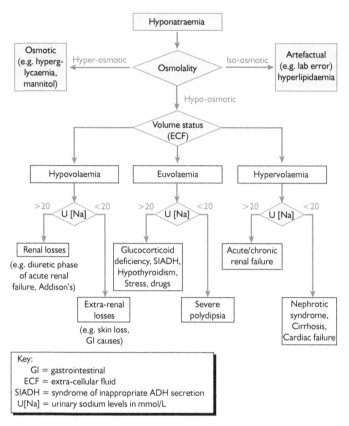

Figure 6.2: Approach to investigating hyponatraemia

Hyponatraemia: causes

◼ Euvolaemic:

• SIADH (syndrome of inappropriate anti-diuretic hormone secretion)

• psychogenic polydipsia

• pure water overload (e.g. iatrogenic – excess administration causing haemodilution)

• severe hypothyroidism.

◼ Volume-depleted:

• fluid losses (vomiting, diarrhoea, high-output drains, burns, fistulae, etc.)

• Addison's disease (adrenal insufficiency)

• diuretics

• renal failure.

◼ Volume-overloaded:

• cardiac failure

• renal failure (nephrotic syndrome)

• liver failure (cirrhosis, hypoalbuminaemia).

Hypernatraemia – high sodium (Na⁺)

Causes

- Dehydration
- Diabetes insipidus
- Excess sodium-containing fluids administered
- Sodium-retaining drugs

Hypokalaemia – low potassium (K⁺)

Causes

- Excess losses (vomiting, diarrhoea, fistulae, stoma)
- Drugs (e.g. diuretics)
- Endocrine disease (e.g. Conn's or Cushing's syndrome)
- Renal disease (e.g. renal tubular acidosis, RTA)

Hyperkalaemia – high potassium (K⁺)

Causes

- Renal failure
- Diabetic ketoacidosis
- Drugs (angiotensin-converting enzyme (ACE)-inhibitors, potassium sparing diuretics such as spironolactone)
- Haemolysis (artefact of venepuncture)
- Endocrine disease (e.g. Addison's disease)
- Rhabdomyolysis

Prostate specific antigen

- PSA is a glycoprotein produced almost exclusively by the cells of the prostate gland.
- Normal value: 0–4 ng/mL ('normal' reference range increases with progressive age).

- The serum PSA reading should always be used in conjunction with digital rectal examination findings and the clinical context; PSA-based screening for prostate cancer remains a contentious issue.

Causes of elevated PSA

- Prostatic malignancy
- Benign prostatic hyperplasia (BPH)
- Infection (prostatitis)
- Other (e.g. exercise, sexual activity)

NB: Digital rectal examination does *not* significantly elevate PSA values.

Calculi

- Calculi (stones) are solid particles that form when components of the urine crystallise along the urinary tract.
- Urinary tract calculi are common (more so in women) and can be extremely painful. Other symptoms include nausea, haematuria and fever/rigors (from secondary infection).
- Most pass spontaneously. Those that do not pass on their own can be removed using procedures such as ureteroscopy or extracorporeal shockwave lithotripsy.
- Composition:
  - calcium based (85%): calcium oxalate (70%), calcium phosphate (15%), calcium urate
  - triple (struvite – magnesium, ammonium, phosphate) (15%)
  - mixed (7%)
  - urate (6%)
  - cysteine (2%).
- Some people are more prone to stone formation than others (there is a genetic component).

Other predisposing factors can also increase the risk of stone formation (e.g. dehydration, infection, hypercalcaemia, hyperparathyroidism, cystinuria, etc.).

Investigation
■ Urinalysis (signs of infection/haematuria).
■ Imaging: plain KUB X-ray (>80% of calculi can be seen on plain radiographs); IVU/P; CTU. Note that CTU is now increasingly replacing IVU in most centres).

Polycystic kidney disease (PKD)

■ This is characterised by the presence of multiple cysts in the kidneys. Cysts can also occur in other organs such as the liver and pancreas.
■ It has a genetic basis, with two main forms:
• autosomal dominant PKD (ADPKD): this has a later onset, with progressive cyst development leading to renal insufficiency and its associated complications. It is caused by mutations of the *PKD1* or *PKD2* genes
• autosomal recessive PKD (ARPKD): this less common disorder often results in early death (either *in utero* or during the first few months of life). It is usually caused by mutations of the *PKHD1* gene.
■ A number of investigative techniques can be used to aid diagnosis. These include:
• imaging (large kidneys)
• genetic testing (for the above mutations).

Nephrotic syndrome

Diagnosis is based on a triad of:
■ proteinuria (>3.5 g/m^2/24 h in adults)
■ hypoabuminaemia (serum albumin <30 g/L)
■ oedema.

Common causes
■ <1 year – congenital nephrotic syndrome
■ 1–40 years – minimal change disease (fusion of podocytes seen on electron microscopy), focal-segmental glomerular sclerosis (FSGS)
■ 40–60 years – glomerulonephritis (especially membranous type), diabetic nephropathy, IgA nephropathy
■ >60 years – amyloidosis

Complications
■ Hyperlipidaemia (increased hepatic production)
■ Acute and chronic renal failure
■ Thromboembolism (can present as recurrent pulmonary embolism)
■ Pleural effusion
■ Hypertension
■ Infection

Urine protein to creatinine ratio
■ Proteinuria is a feature of a number of renal pathologies.
■ Traditionally, a 24h urine collection is used to measure the concentration of protein excreted over a fixed time.
■ However, these are inconvenient for patients and can also be inaccurate.
■ The urine protein:creatinine ratio is a more convenient method of estimating the 24h protein excretion, and hence the degree of proteinuria.
■ This is based on the principle that creatinine excretion (dependent on

body weight) remains fairly constant throughout the day (not dependent on urine flow rate).

■ The protein:creatinine ratio/100 is approximately equal to the 24 h protein collection level (e.g. protein:creatinine ration of 2 ≈ 0.02 g/24 h).

■ Ratios:

• <2 mg/mmol = normal

• 20–50 mg/mmol = slightly elevated, but usually indicates no serious disease (provided estimated GFR (eGFR) is normal). Requires further investigation in patients with diabetes mellitus

• 50–300 mg/mmol = high – requires further investigation

• >300 mg/mmol = nephrotic syndrome range.

NB: In the USA, different units (mg/dL) are used. For example, a urinary protein of 85 mg/dL and urinary creatinine of 25 mg/dL, gives a ratio = 85/25 = 3.4 (i.e. equivalent to roughly 3.4 g protein excretion over 24 h. With this scale, <0.5 = normal (children); <0.2 = normal (adults); >3.5 = high, e.g. in the 'nephrotic range'.

Nephritic syndrome (glomerulonephritis)

This is a disorder of glomeruli, characterised by:

■ haematuria (+/– red cell casts)

■ +/– oedema

■ +/– hypertension.

The most accurate diagnosis is made with histology (renal biopsy).

Types

■ Post-infective:

• usually a *streptococcal* throat infection

• can also have other bacterial, viral or parasitic aetiologies

• raised anti-streptolysin O (ASO) titres

• commonly between ages 2 and 14 years.

■ Membranous (membrano-proliferative).

■ IgA nephropathy (Berger's disease):

• commonest cause worldwide

• young patients, rapid recovery between episodes

• often progressive

• a common cause of end-stage renal failure.

■ Henoch-Schönlein purpura:

• variant of IgA nephropathy, usually presents in children

• large-joint polyarthritis, purpuric rash of extensor surfaces, abdominal symptoms.

■ Mesangio-capillary:

• Type 1 = subendothelial deposits

• Type 2 = intramembranous deposits.

■ Proliferative.

■ Goodpasture's syndrome:

• anti-glomerular basement membrane antibodies.

■ Wegener's granulomatosis:

• untreated, this carries a 90% mortality at 1 year.

■ Rapidly progressive:

• variant of the above characterised by end-stage renal failure occurring in weeks to months

• glomerular basement membrane and anti-neutrophil cytoplasmic antibody (ANCA) positive renal disease are usually the most rapidly progressive.

Presentation

Features can include any of the following.

- Asymptomatic (e.g. through a screening investigation such as for an insurance company medical test)
- 'Classic' signs (haematuria, proteinuria, hypertension)
- Nephrotic syndrome
- Renal failure
- Systemic complications (e.g. pulmonary symptoms, rash, joint pains, etc.)

Acute versus chronic renal failure

Glomerular filtration rate (GFR)

- GFR is essentially a measurement of the rate of the kidney's ability to clear waste from the plasma compartment (i.e. the volume of plasma ultrafiltrate produced by the glomeruli, per unit time).
- The 'normal' range is lower in certain ethnic groups and with renal disease.
- While renal function is usually estimated using plasma urea, creatinine and electrolyte measurements, these may often be 'normal' in the early stages of renal disease.

Creatinine-based GFR estimates
- A number of formulae exist to calculate an estimate of the creatinine clearance, and hence an estimate of the GFR (eGFR).

MDRD
- The abbreviated (4-variable) modification of diet in renal disease (MDRD) formula determines the eGFR based on the patient's age, sex, and serum creati-

nine. More accurate versions of this formula also incorporate other variables, such as serum albumin and the 'blood urea nitrogen' measurement (more commonly used in the USA).

$$eGFR\,(mL/min) = 32788 \times \\ \text{serum creatinine}\,(\mu mol/L)^{-1.154} \times \\ age^{-0.203} \times [1.21\,\text{if black}] \times \\ [0.742\,\text{if female}]$$

Cockcroft-Gault
- The Cockcroft-Gault equation is perhaps a more well known creatinine-based formula for estimating GFR:

$$\text{Creatinine clearance}\,(mL/min) = \\ \frac{(140 - age) \times weight\,(kg)\,(\times\,constant)}{72 \times serum\,creatinine\,(\mu mol/L)}$$

NB: constant = 1.23 (male), 1.04 (female).
Normal GFR = usually >90 mL/min (although measurements >60 (female) and >70 (male) are often accepted as normal in most patients).

Creatinine clearance
- This is the volume of plasma cleared of creatinine, per unit time.
- This can be used to estimate the GFR, as creatinine is freely filtered at the glomerulus and is not reabsorbed (however, unlike inulin, there can be some secretion in the tubules, hence creatinine clearance usually over-estimates GFR).
- Plasma creatinine is therefore inversely proportional to GFR (although note that this is a non-linear relationship).
- Determining the urinary creatinine and urinary flow rates requires a 24 h urine collection.

$$\text{Creatinine clearance (mL/min)} = \frac{[\text{Urine creatinine conc.] (mmol/L)} \times \text{Urine flow rate (mL/min)}}{[\text{Plasma creatinine conc.] (mmol/L)}}$$

Tracer-based methods of measuring GFR

■ While GFR is usually estimated by calculating the creatinine clearance, it can be more specifically determined by measuring the clearance of a number of substances.

■ This is more commonly used in research settings.

■ Traditionally, inulin clearance is described. As inulin is freely filtered (neither reabsorbed nor secreted by the kidney) its excretion rate is directly proportional to the GFR.

■ As filtered inulin = excreted inulin:

$$GFR = \frac{Urinary_{in} \times volume}{Plasma_{in}}$$

NB: Urinary clearance is measured in mL/min.

■ 51 Chromium EDTA, a radioactive isotope administered IV, can also be used to determine GFR. However, this is a time-consuming and expensive process, so it is usually reserved for certain specialised situations (e.g. when a very accurate measurement of GFR is required for calculating chemotherapy dose).

Acute renal failure

■ This is a significant deterioration in renal function occurring over hours to days, characterised by a raised plasma urea and creatinine.

■ In 'pre-renal' causes, the kidneys attempt to retain salt and water.

■ The reverse is true in 'renal' causes.

■ The aim of treatment is to prevent acute tubular necrosis (ATN, reversible) from progressing to acute cortical necrosis (permanent). The only treatment for ATN, if it occurs, is expectant (i.e. time).

	Pre-renal	ATN
Urine Na (mmol/L)	<20	>40
Urine osmolarity (mosm/L)	>500	<350
Urine/plasma urea	<8	<3
Urine/plasma creatinine	<40	<20
Fractional Na excretion (%)	<1	<2

Chronic renal failure

■ This is the substantial, irreversible and usually long-standing loss of renal function.

■ Chronic kidney disease (CKD) is now classified into five stages (by the UK Renal Association and Royal College of Physicians).

Stage 1: Normal GFR or GFR of >90 mL/min with evidence of renal disease (e.g. proteinuria for polycystic kidney disease, etc.). Need to have kidney function tested every 12 months. Very common.

Stage 2: Mild impairment of GFR (between 60 and 89 mL/min) and evidence of renal disease. Should have renal function checked every 12 months.

Stage 3: Moderate impairment of GFR (between 30 and 59 mL/min). Renal function should be tested every 6–12 months, depending on clinical stability. Patients may require specialist input at this stage.

Stage 4: Severe impairment of GFR (between 15 and 29 mL/min). Renal function should be tested every 3–6 months.

Stage 5: Established renal failure (ERF), GFR <15 mL/min. Patients usually require dialysis at this stage (and are usually under specialist care).

Adapted from http://www.renal.org/CKDguide/full/Conciseguid 141205.pdf

Evidence of chronic renal disease includes:

- persistent microalbuminuria
- persistent proteinuria
- persistent haematuria
- structural abnormalities.

Anion gap

- This measurement can be used to help investigate the various causes of metabolic acidosis.
- The 'gap' is made up of unmeasured ions such as phosphate, sulphate and lactate.
- It is calculated as follows:

$$\text{Anion gap} = (Na^+ + K^+) - (Cl^- + HCO_3^-)$$

Normal range: 4–17 mmol/L

High

- Any condition with reduced clearance or excess production of any unmeasured anions (e.g. diabetic ketoacidosis, lactic acidosis, ethanol excess)

Low

- Hyperalbuminaemia
- Liver disease
- Paraproteinaemias

Chapter 7
NEUROLOGY

Introduction

A detailed history and examination are the most important elements of characterising a neurological disorder and will often allow diagnosis with anatomical localisation of the neuropathological process. As with all specialties, investigation can play an important role in reaching the diagnosis and in guiding management. While this chapter is by no means exhaustive, we have presented a few different approaches to investigating some common neurological disorders. Imaging (especially CT or MRI scanning) is one of the most commonly used modalities for investigating neurological pathology; although this is discussed in more depth in Chapter 15, we have outlined some of the indications of neurological imaging here.

Topics covered
- Approach to neurological localisation
- Neurological examination
- Cranial nerves
- Key neurological investigations
- Approach to neurological disorders

Approach to neurological localisation

- Common neurological conditions typically have distinctive clinical features often related to the anatomical site of the pathological process.
- In assessing a neurological disorder it may therefore be helpful to consider broad divisions according to anatomical site.
- Central nervous system (CNS):
- brain, e.g. encephalopathies, dementias, stroke
- basal ganglia and cerebellum, e.g. parkinsonism
- brainstem, e.g. demyelination
- spinal cord, e.g. central disc prolapse.
- Peripheral nervous system (PNS):
- nerve roots, e.g. sciatica
- peripheral nerves, e.g. alcoholic neuropathies, carpal tunnel syndrome
- neuromuscular junction (NMJ), e.g. myasthenia gravis
- muscle, e.g. dermatomyositis.

Central pathology
- Pathology affecting the brain may lead to motor or sensory symptoms/

The hands-on guide to data interpretation. By S. Abraham, K. Kulkarni, R. Madhu and D. Provan. Published 2010 by Blackwell Publishing Ltd.

signs, as well as other features including an alteration in conscious level, cognitive dysfunction, seizures, speech disturbance and visual field defects.

■ Pathology affecting the basal ganglia typically cause movement disorders, e.g. Parkinsonism, chorea. The hallmark of cerebellar disorders is ataxia.

■ Pathology affecting the brainstem typically results in symptoms and signs of cranial nerve pathology.

■ Pathology affecting the spinal cord classically presents with paraplegia or quadriplegia with sphincter disturbance (urinary retention) and a sensory level.

Peripheral pathology

■ Peripheral nerve disorders may produce a lower motor neuron weakness with wasting/fasciculation, depressed/absent reflexes and reduced tone with a distal to proximal progression. Sensory disturbance is typically a 'glove and stocking' loss.

■ NMJ and muscle disorders often cause proximal weakness with no sensory disturbance. NMJ disorders are characterised by fatigability.

Summary

■ The interpretation of any neurological investigation should be in the context of the clinical findings.

■ Investigations may allow both refinement of the anatomical localisation as well as determining the nature of the neurological disorder.

■ Important neurological investigations include:

• cerebrospinal fluid (CSF) analysis
• nerve conduction studies (NCS) and electromyelography (EMG)
• evoked potentials
• electroencephalogram (EEG)

• computed tomography (CT)/ magnetic resonance imaging (MRI)/ angiography.

Neurological examination

Assessment of muscle strength

■ Weakness is an important symptom/ sign.

■ The pattern of weakness and mode of onset may provide clues to aetiology, e.g. an acute hemiplegia is suggestive of a stroke; progressive paraplegia may indicate a chronic spinal cord pathology.

■ The Medical Research Council (MRC) grading of muscle strength provides an objective measure to monitor a patent's weakness.

MRC grading of muscle strength

This scale can be used for quantitatively grading limb muscle power. Maximum ('best') score = 5.

0 = complete paralysis (no contraction)
1 = flicker of contraction
2 = active movement if gravity excluded
3 = active movement against gravity
4 = moderate power movement against resistance
5 = normal power

Voluntary muscle control is mediated through the pyramidal system. The upper motor neuron (UMN) originates in the motor cortex and runs in the corticospinal tracts to synapse with lower motor neurons (LMN) in the anterior horn of the spinal cord. It is particularly helpful to consider weakness as upper motor neuron or lower motor neuron in trying to determine aetiology.

Lesions of the UMN and LMN each have a characteristic set of associated signs and symptoms. The table below summarises the key differences.

Feature	UMN	LMN
Definition	Above level of anterior horn (e.g. spinal tracts, internal capsule)	Below level of anterior horn (e.g. peripheral nerve)
Muscle wasting	Little/none	Marked
Fasciculations	None	May be present
Tone	Increased (hypertonia)	Reduced (hypotonia)
Clonus	Can be present (>3 beats)	Absent (<3 beats)
Weakness	Predominantly upper limb flexors/lower limb extensors ('pyramidal weakness')	Weakness may be localised to peripheral nerve or root territory or more pronounced distally
Reflexes	Hyper-reflexia	Hypo-reflexia
Plantar reflex	Up going (Babinski +ve)	Down going

Reflexes

■ Assessment of reflexes is useful to help localise lesions and in distinguishing upper and lower motor neuron disorders.

■ Note that hyper-reflexia can also occur when patients are anxious or when they are trying to assist the examiner with reflex testing.

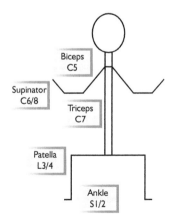

Figure 7.1: Spinal roots associated with some important reflexes

Dermatomes

A dermatome is a region of skin innervated by a single dorsal spinal nerve root.

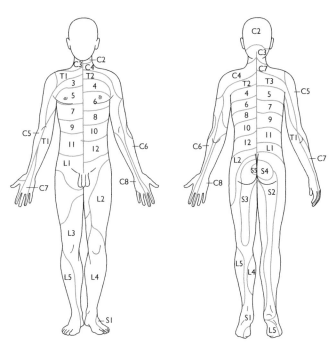

Figure 7.2: Distribution of dermatomes

Upper limb: sensory distribution

The wrist and hand are primarily inner-vated by three peripheral nerves: the median, the ulnar and the radial (all branches of the brachial plexus).

Median nerve distribution
(C6, C7, C8 and T1)
Ulnar nerve distribution
(C8, T1)
Radial nerve distribution
(C5, C6, C7, C8 and T1)
Medial brachial cutaneous
nerve of arm and forearm

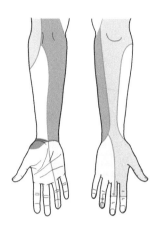

Figure 7.3: Upper limb sensory nerve distribution

Lower limb: sensory distribution

Nerve	Origin	Distribution
Lateral femoral cutaneous	L2,3	sensory: lateral side of thigh
Femoral	L2,3,4	motor: anterior thigh muscles sensory: anterior thigh and medial half (lower leg)
Obturator	L2,3,4	motor: thigh and knee adductors sensory: proximal medial thigh
Superior gluteal	L4,5; S1	motor: gluteus medius and minimus, tensor fasciae latae
Inferior gluteal	L5; S1,2	motor: gluteus maximus
Posterior femoral cutaneous	S1,2,3	sensory: posterior thigh
Pudendal	S2,3,4	sensory: external genitalia, perineum, anus

(Continued)

(Continued)

Nerve	Origin	Distribution
Sciatic	L4,5; S1,2,3	motor/sensory: (tibial, peroneal branches)
	tibial branch	motor: (superficial and deep branches) sensory: proximal lateral lower leg (and superficial and deep branches)
	common peroneal	motor: hamstring muscles, posterior compartment of lower leg sensory: distal posterior lower leg
	superficial peroneal	motor: lateral compartment of lower leg sensory: distal anterior lower leg
	deep peroneal	motor: anterior compartment of lower leg sensory: part of dorsal foot

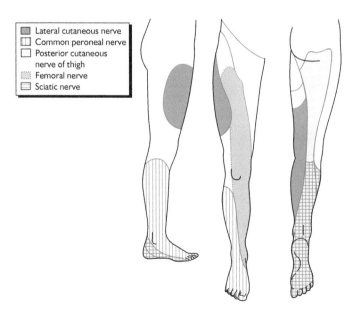

■ Lateral cutaneous nerve
▥ Common peroneal nerve
☐ Posterior cutaneous nerve of thigh
▨ Femoral nerve
▤ Sciatic nerve

Figure 7.4: Lower limb sensory nerve distribution

Cranial nerves

Lesions of each cranial nerve can lead to characteristic focal neurological signs.

I	Olfactory	Anomie (change in smell, also associated with change in taste)
II	Optic	Visual loss – AFRO: **A**cuity, **F**ields, **R**eflexes, **O**phthalmoscopy (Fundoscopy)
III	Oculomotor	Eye deviates down and out Impaired pupillary/accommodation reflexes
IV	Trochlear	Diplopia Lateral deviation of eye
V	Trigeminal	Facial anaesthesia (in distribution of ophthalmic, maxillary or mandibular divisions) Weakness of mastication
VI	Abducens	Medial eye deviation
VII	Facial	Impaired facial expression (e.g. inability to 'puff out cheeks' or 'raise eyebrows', etc.) Hyperacusis Loss of taste (anterior 2/3rd of tongue) Dry mouth, loss of lacrimation
VIII	Vestibulocochlear	Vertigo, disequilibrium, nystagmus, hearing loss
IX	Glossopharyngeal	Impaired taste (posterior 1/3rd of tongue) . Impaired gag reflex Uvular deviation (away from side of lesion)
X	Vagus	Dysphagia Hoarseness of voice Impaired cough reflex Impaired taste
XI	Accessory	Head turning/shoulder shrugging weakness
XII	Hypoglossal	Fasciculation/atrophy of tongue muscles Deviation on protrusion (towards side of lesion)

Cranial nerve reflexes

Reflex	Sensory (Afferent)	Motor (Efferent)
Pupil: light/accommodation	II	III
Jaw jerk	V	V
Corneal	V	VII
Vestibulo-ocular	VIII	III, IV, VI +
Gag	IX	X

Visual fields

Lesions of the optic nerve (II) can lead to impairment of the visual field. The type of visual loss varies depending on where along the tract the lesion is.

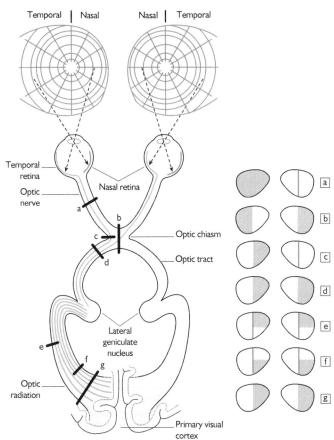

A – left-sided blindness
B – bitemporal hemianopia
C – left nasal hemianopia
D – homonymous hemianopia
E – homonymous quadrantinopia
F – homonymous hemianopia
G – binasal hemianopia

Figure 7.5: Visual fields

NB: Further details about the assessment of visual fields and acuity can be found in Chapter 11.

Eye movement

A number of muscles are involved in eye movement. These are innervated by the oculomotor (III), trochlear (IV) and abducens (VI) cranial nerves.

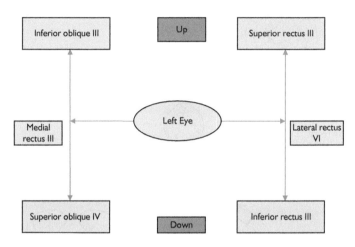

Key:
III (occulomotor = all, except those innervated by IV & VI)
IV (trochlear) = **S**uperior **O**blique,
VI (occulomotor) = **L**ateral **R**ectus

('LR6, SO4')

Figure 7.6: Eye muscles and their movements

Hearing

Rinne and Weber tests
Weber test

■ This is used to detect unilateral conductive hearing loss.

■ A struck tuning fork (256/512 Hz) placed on the midline (e.g. middle of the forehead) is normally heard at equal volume in both ears.

■ If there is a conductive hearing loss in one ear, the sound localises (i.e. is heard loudest) in the affected ear.

■ If there is sensorineural hearing loss in one ear, the sound localises to the other (normal) ear.

Rinne test

■ In conjunction with the Weber test, this can be used to screen for a sensorineural hearing loss.

A struck tuning fork is placed on the mastoid process until sound is no longer heard. The tuning fork is then placed approximately 3 inches outside the ear.

If there is normal hearing, air conduction (AC) is better than bone conduction (BC) – a positive Rinne.

BC is better than AC (negative Rinne) if there is conductive or sensorineural hearing loss in the ear tested.

Example: sensorineural hearing loss in left ear

Weber test: sound will be heard loudest in the right ear, meaning either: (a) a conductive hearing loss on the right, or (b) a sensorineural hearing loss on the left.

The Rinne test: on the left side, BC > AC (abnormal). On the right side AC > BC (normal). As the Weber test has already indicated that there is no conductive hearing loss on the left, this localises the source of the problem as a sensorineural hearing loss on the left.

Audiogram

While Rinne's and Weber's tests are helpful screening tests, an audiogram can provide a more quantitative assessment of an individuals hearing.

Characteristic patterns can provide clues as to the aetiology of any hearing loss (e.g. to distinguish between conductive, sensorineural and age-related hearing loss).

Conductive versus sensorineural hearing loss
Conductive deafness

This includes anything that affects the normal conduction of sound through the outer and middle ear.

This can be due to damage or obstruction to the ear canal, ear drum (tympanic membrane) or the ossicles, i.e. due to impaired air or bone conduction.

Common causes include impacted ear wax (cerumen) or infection (e.g. otitis externa/media).

The audiogram shows air conduction worse than bone conduction (Figure 7.7).

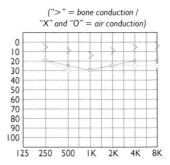

(">" = bone conduction / "X" and "O" = air conduction)

Figure 7.7: Audiogram showing conductive hearing loss

Sensorineural deafness

This is permanent hearing loss, resulting from damage to the inner ear (cochlea and associated structures) through to the auditory nerve.

Causes include presbycusis (see below), noise exposure, tumours (e.g. acoustic neuroma), drugs, infection (e.g. measles, mumps) and Ménière's disease.

The audiogram shows both, air and bone conduction to be similarly impaired (Figure 7.8).

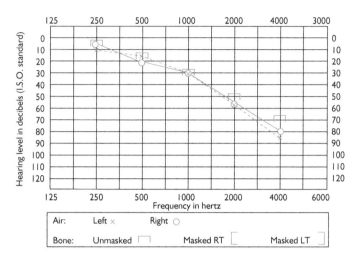

An example of a mild to severe sensorineural hearing loss in both ears.

Figure 7.8: Audiogram showing sensorineural hearing loss

Age-related deafness (presbycusis)

■ This is a feature of normal ageing and is a form of sensorineural hearing loss.

■ The audiogram shows a characteristic pattern of high-frequency sensorineural hearing loss (hence air and bone conduction are similarly affected) (Figure 7.9).

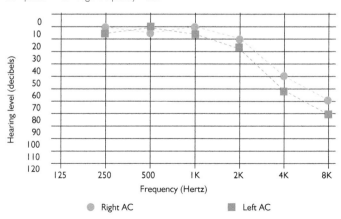

Figure 7.9: Audiogram showing presbycusis

Key neurological investigations

Neurological imaging

Imaging is a key investigative modality for many neurological disorders. Some modalities include the following.

Computed tomography (CT)

■ Benefits: fast, cheap, reliable.
■ Indications:
• current imaging modality of choice in assessment of acute stroke
• acute haemorrhage including subarachnoid haemorrhage
• bone imaging (acute trauma, fractures)
• when MRI is contraindicated.
■ Contrast enhancement is used to opacify blood vessels:
• CT-venogram is useful for investigating cerebral venous sinus thrombosis
• CT-angiograms allow investigation of the cerebrovascular system.

Magnetic resonance imaging (MRI)

■ High resolution of soft tissues and therefore imaging modality of choice in many cases.
■ Many different protocols available and interpretation can be complex, for example:
• T1 – tissue discrimination and with contrast agents (gadolinium) to identify enhancing lesions
• T2 – very sensitive to increased water and so visualise oedema
• STIR (short tau inversion recovery) – fat-suppressed sequence with high sensitivity for the study of skeletal conditions (e.g. tumours, or infections such as tuberculosis and discitis)

• FLAIR (fluid attenuated inversion recovery) – CSF signal suppressed, allowing subtle T2 abnormalities to be visible
• DWI (diffusion weighted imaging) – sensitive to restricted water diffusion as seen in cytotoxic oedema
• Gradient-echo - blood products, iron, calcium more readily seen.
■ MR angiography can be used to image cerebrovascular system.

X-ray

A number of types of X-ray can be of use in investigating neurological pathology, including chest X-ray (e.g. for investigating lung malignancies associated with focal neurological signs), skull (infrequently used, e.g. for sinuses, pituitary fossa) and spine (commonly used in the trauma setting to visualise the cervical spine).
■ Ultrasound: Doppler/duplex ultrasound is commonly used to investigate vascular carotid artery disease (e.g. post transient ischaemic attack or stroke).
■ Arteriography: the gold standard for imaging cerebrovascular system for example in the investigation of aneurysms and arteriovenous malformations.
■ Isotope scanning: positron emission tomography (PET) and single photon emission CT (SPECT) can be used to visualise blood flow and metabolic activity (e.g. in the investigation of seizures or tumours).
See Chapter 15 for more details.

Cerebrospinal fluid (CSF) analysis

■ The analysis of CSF, obtained via a lumbar puncture (LP), is useful in the diagnosis of a number of conditions, including meningitis and subarachnoid haemorrhage.

■ Care must be taken not to perform a LP if increased intracranial pressure is suspected (e.g. focal neurology with depressed conscious level, papilloedema)*, bleeding diathesis or infection at the puncture site.

*A CT must be performed to assess risk of herniation (e.g. midline shift, obliteration of 4th ventricle).

■ Always remember to take a corresponding venous blood sample in order to compare glucose and oligoclonal bands.

	Usual	Viral meningitis	Bacterial meningitis	Tuberculosis meningitis
Appearance	Clear	Clear/turbid	Turbid	Viscous
Differential cell type	Very few mononuclear cells	10–100 mm^3 mononuclear cells	200–300 mm^3 polymorph cells	100–300 mm^3 mononuclear cells. Up to 200 mm^3 polymorph cells
Protein	0.2–0.4 g/L	0.4–0.8 g/L	0.5–2.0 g/L	0.5–3.0 g/L
Glucose	$\frac{2}{3}$–$\frac{1}{2}$ of blood glucose	>$\frac{1}{2}$ blood glucose	<$\frac{1}{2}$ of blood glucose	<$\frac{1}{2}$ of blood glucose

Other findings

■ Xanthochromia (usually bilirubin from broken-down haemoglobin, i.e. subarachnoid haemorrhage (SAH)). Can also be seen with high levels of CSF proteins (e.g. chronic inflammatory demyelinating polyneuropathy, spinal block).

■ Oligoclonal bands = multiple sclerosis (also subacute sclerosing panencephalitis, Guillain-Barré syndrome, Lyme disease, neurosyphillis). NB: need to compare presence of bands in CSF and serum; presence in CSF only indicates CNS pathology.

■ Raised protein = meningitis, abscess, connective tissue diseases, Guillain-Barré syndrome.

■ Gram stain = undertaken on a sediment of the CSF and is positive in the majority of cases of bacterial meningitis. Culture can also be performed on samples, as can be other stains (e.g. Ziehl Neelson stain for acid-fast bacilli with Mycobacterium tuberculosis infection).

■ Polymerase chain reaction (PCR): This has high sensitivity, particularly in the investigation of viral and tuberculous meningitis.

Conditions investigated by lumbar puncture (LP)

■ Meningitis.

■ Subarachnoid haemorrhage (SAH):

- Xanthochromia (a yellowish discolouration) can be detected from 12 h and for up to 2 weeks after the event.
- blood in all of the sample bottles (as opposed to a traumatic tap in which blood is detected in the first bottle, but subsequent sample bottles are clearer).
- Labs increasingly provide a 'bilirubin/oxyhaemoglobin profile':
– RBC in CSF lyse after 2–12 h releasing oxyhaemoglobin
– in vivo, oxyhaemoglobin is gradually converted to bilirubin
– typically in SAH, bilirubin and oxyhaemoglobin will be raised.

Demyelinating disease

■ Immunoglobulins can be detected in the CSF with conditions such as multiple sclerosis (characteristic 'oligoclonal bands').

■ Raised IgG can also be found with other conditions such as neurosyphillis, Guillain-Barré syndrome, systemic lupus erythematosus, etc.

■ Serum versus CSF oligoclonal bands: oligoclonal bands in the CSF but not in the serum indicate central nervous system production.

Electromyography (EMG)

■ This investigation involves the recording of muscle action potentials after electrical stimulation.

■ Both needle electrodes and surface recordings can be used.

■ EMG is useful in the investigation of myopathic disorders (muscle wasting/weakness), including: myasthenia gravis, polymyositis, motor neurone disease or myotonic dystrophy. Generalised muscle damage results in a characteristic pattern of short, polyphasic potentials. However, the specific cause cannot usually be identified.

■ EMG can also be used to help diagnose neuropathies (e.g. axonal versus demyelinating), with the resting 'fibrillation' activity being replaced by features such as 'fasciculations' or 'positive sharp waves' with denervation.

■ 'Repetitive stimulation' is a superficial recording technique that can be used to investigate myasthenia gravis. In this, repeated supra-maximal nerve stimulation results in a decreasing response. However, this test is often overlooked in favour of single fibre EMG recordings and measurement of acetylcholine receptor antibody estimation.

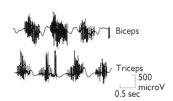

Figure 7.10: EMG recordings from the upper limb

Nerve conduction studies

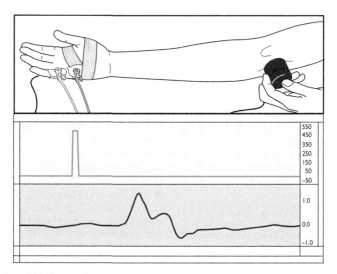

Figure 7.11: Nerve conduction study

■ These measure the conduction of electrical impulses along motor and sensory nerves. An electrical stimulus is used to trigger a response in a peripheral nerve, which is then recorded.

■ Recordings include the nerve conduction velocity, latency (time for impulse to travel from stimulation site to recording site) and amplitude of response.

■ These parameters depend on the nerve fibre type, diameter and myelination. Large myelinated fibres such as the alpha motor nerves have the fastest conduction velocities.

■ Nerve conduction studies consist of several components, including:

• motor (recording from a muscle supplied by a nerve)

• sensory (recording from the sensory aspect of a nerve)

• F-wave (uses supramaximal stimulation to record action potentials from a muscle supplied by a nerve, i.e. conduction velocity of nerve between muscle and spinal cord).

■ They can be of use in a range of pathologies, for example focal entrapment neuropathies, such as carpal tunnel syndrome (slowing of median nerve latencies), or more generalised degenerative neuropathies (e.g. alcoholic/ diabetic).

■ Broadly speaking, neuropathic abnormalities can be classified into:

• axonopathy, e.g. alcoholic neuropathy

• demyelination, e.g. Guillain-Barré syndrome.

■ Demyelinating neuropathies may be amenable to treatment with IV immunoglobulins, plasmapheresis or immune modulating drugs (e.g. steroids).

	Axonopathy	Demyelination
Nerve conduction velocity	Preserved or slightly reduced	Significantly reduced
Conduction block	Not present	Present
Distal motor latency	Normal or slightly prolonged	Prolonged
Amplitude of compound muscle action potential (CMAP)	Small	Normal (reduced if conduction block)
Sensory responses	Small	Small
Examples of associated conditions	Alcoholic neuropathy	Guillain-Barré syndrome, chronic inflammatory demyelinating neuropathy

Muscle and nerve biopsy

Muscle biopsy

■ This can be used to investigate certain neuromuscular pathologies, e.g. dystrophy, myositis, myopathy, etc.

■ Biopsy samples are taken by either percutaneous needle or open biopsy, and are histologically examined for the presence of abnormal cells (e.g. inflammatory) as well as other features such as change in fibre size/shape. Special stains can be used to examine the muscle tissue for the presence of muscle enzymes (e.g. phosphorylase).

Nerve biopsy

■ This is a similar procedure, performed under local anaesthetic, used to obtain a sample of nerve tissue for histological examination.

■ Nerves more commonly biopsied include the sural nerve, the superficial radial nerve and the ulnar nerve. Samples can be full or partial thickness.

■ Biopsies are of benefit when they can be used to diagnose and assess the severity of potentially treatable neuropathies. These include:
• immune-mediated neuropathies (e.g. vasculitis, sarcoidosis)
• other treatable neuropathies (e.g. CMV neuritis, leprosy).

■ Biopsies can also be used to distinguish between demyelination and axonal degeneration.

Evoked potentials (EP)

Visual evoked potentials (VEP)

■ This involves the eye being stimulated using a variety of visual stimuli patterns, and responses being recorded over the occipital cortex.

■ Stimuli can include flashes or checkerboard patterns.

■ The speed of neural response (latency) and the strength or amplitude of the positive occipital cortical potential (the response) are recorded. The latency is usually about 100 ms ('P100').

■ This investigation is often used to investigate multiple sclerosis, in which there is usually a delayed response (delay in P100) secondary to optic nerve demyelination. Other causes include tumours compressing the optic nerve, vitamin B12 deficiency and inflammation (e.g. secondary to conditions such as sarcoid).

Sensory evoked potentials (SEP)

■ These are recordings taken over the spinal cord in response to peripheral skin stimulation.

■ They can be used to measure conduction through nerve plexi, e.g. the brachial or lumbar plexus, as well as the central conduction pathways.

Brainstem sensory evoked potentials (BSEP)

■ These can be used to record potentials from the acoustic nerve (wave I), cochlear and olivary nuclei (II and III), lateral lemniscus (IV), inferior colliculus (V) and subcortical structures (VI and VII).

■ They can be used to investigate acoustic neuromas and other brainstem lesion (with abnormalities being found in conditions such as multiple sclerosis, stroke, head injury, tumours, etc.).

Electroencephalography (EEG)

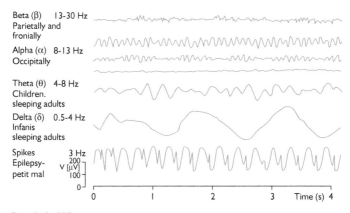

Beta (β) 13-30 Hz
Parietally and
fronially

Alpha (α) 8-13 Hz
Occipitally

Theta (θ) 4-8 Hz
Children.
sleeping adults

Delta (δ) 0.5-4 Hz
Infanis
sleeping adults

Spikes 3 Hz
Epilepsy-
petit mal

V [μV] 200 / 100 / 0

0   1   2   3   Time (s) 4

Figure 7.12: EEG patterns

■ This involves recording of the low-amplitude electrical activity of the brain, using scalp electrodes.

■ The signals recorded reflect the voltage differences in the global activity of a range of neurones.

■ EEG plays a role in the management of a number of conditions, including:
• epilepsy (certain types of seizure activity demonstrating characteristic complex patterns, e.g. '3Hz spike and wave' in absence seizures)
• sleep disorders
• coma states.

■ Recording usually takes place with eyes open, eyes closed, and during hyperventilation and photic stimulation (to enhance abnormalities and induce paroxysmal disturbances).

■ Recordings can sometimes be undertaken under certain special conditions, e.g. during sleep or in the ambulatory setting.

The different waves of an EEG

■ Awake: beta waves (low voltage, high frequency ≥30 Hz).
■ Drowsy: alpha waves (8–12 Hz).
■ Stage 1 sleep: theta waves (3–7 Hz).
■ Stage 2 sleep: sleep spindles & K complexes (12–14 Hz).
■ Stage 3/4 sleep (deep): delta waves (0.5–4 Hz).
■ REM sleep: beta waves.

Note that artefacts may be present due to movement (e.g. tremor), sweating or electrical interference from nearby equipment.

EEG features in different disorders

■ Encephalitis: focal/generalised slow rhythms, occasional large-amplitude complexes or superimposed paroxysmal discharges (features of encephalitis as well as other severe brain damage, e.g. anoxic/hypoglycaemic injury).

■ Degenerative disorders: low-amplitude EEG with prominent fast activity (e.g. in Huntington's). Periodic complexes (e.g. in Creutzfeldt-Jakob Disease, CJD). Mild slowing (e.g. early Alzheimer's).

■ Metabolic disorders: increased fast activity (e.g. drugs – benzodiazepines). Slowing of alpha activity and replacement by theta/delta activity (e.g. drug intoxication).

■ Epilepsy: please see section below.

Brain biopsy

■ This procedure can be used to obtain a definitive diagnose of certain pathologies, such as tumours, and less commonly for degenerative conditions and inflammatory disorders (e.g. vasculitis).

■ This procedure is usually image guided (by CT or MRI).

■ A stereotactic biopsy involves the use of a frame fixed to the skull. Combined with imaging, this allows the biopsy site to be accurately determined, leading to a more precise needle approach.

■ Histopathology of the samples may then allow a tissue diagnosis.

Other tests

Several blood or urine-based tests can be of particular use when investigating neurological disease. They include the following.

■ Full blood count: a macrocytic anaemic is suggestive of vitamin B12 deficiency, which can be a cause of peripheral neuropathy. Macrocytosis can also be suggestive of excess alcohol intake (a cause of neuropathy, precise mechanism remains unclear).

■ Erythrocyte sedimentation rate (ESR): although a crude marker of general inflammation, a very high ESR can suggest pathologies such as a vasculitic process (e.g. the cause of the presenting headache), mononeuritis multiplex or stroke, etc.

■ Liver function tests (LFTs): these can be deranged with excess alcohol intake.

■ Blood culture/viral serology: useful in detecting the presence of an infective agent (e.g. as the cause of meningitis/encephalitis).

■ Anticonvulsant levels: these can be used to help determine whether drug therapy is in the therapeutic (or toxic) range. Note, however, that blood levels should be assessed in conjunction with the clinical status – there can often be a tendency to unnecessarily adjust the dose to treat the number rather than the patient.

■ Toxicology screen: this can be undertaken with both serum and urine samples and can be used to detect levels of a range of substances including alcohol and drugs (prescription and illicit).

■ Auto-antibodies: some common uses of auto-antibodies have been described elsewhere in this chapter (e.g. myasthenia gravis).

■ Creatine kinase (CK):
• this rises with muscle damage/necrosis ('normal' levels are usually <100 IU). Values can rise with exertion, so samples should ideally be taken after rest
• causes of elevated levels include: muscle trauma, muscular dystrophies (e.g. Becker/Duchenne), drug-related myopathy (e.g. alcoholic), inflammatory myopathies (e.g. polymyositis), etc.

■ Myoglobinuria:
• this is the presence of myoglobin in the urine
• it is another marker of muscle necrosis (rhabdomyolysis), e.g. secondary to trauma

• excessive myoglobin can lead to tubular necrosis and acute renal failure.

Approach to neurological disorders

Assessment of consciousness, awareness and confusion

■ Acute confusional states are characterised by impaired cognition and attention, commonly with a fluctuating level of consciousness.

■ The commonest causes of acute confusion are systemic/metabolic disorders:
• respiratory, hepatic, renal dysfunction
• toxins, drugs, alcohol
• electrolyte/metabolite imbalance – sodium, calcium, magnesium, glucose
• systemic sepsis
• thyroid/adrenal dysfunction.

■ Important neurological causes include:
• CNS infection, e.g. meningitis, HSV encephalitis
• seizures/post-ictal
• cerebrovascular lesions
• CNS inflammation, e.g. neurosarcoid.

■ The approach to a confused patient will consist of:
• obtaining a good collateral history
• a general and neurological examination
• an assessment of the level of consciousness and neuropsychological impairments.

■ Investigations should seek to exclude systemic disorders:

- e.g. FBC, ESR/CRP, LFT, U/E, TFT, Ca, Mg
- septic screen (MSU, blood cultures, etc.)
- CXR, ECG.

■ Appropriate neurological investigations include:
- CT/MRI – structural lesion, stroke, raised ICP
- CSF – ?CNS infection
- EEG – ?seizures *NB:* slow wave activity is a non-specific feature of encephalopathy.

AVPU scale

This is a cruder but quick scale often used in emergency settings to obtain a basic assessment of the patient's status.

The patient responds to:

Alert
Voice
Pain
Unresponsive

Glasgow Coma Scale (GCS)

■ This is an objective system for assessing three key components of an individual's global response status.

■ The principle is that by being standardised, scores can be compared over time, and between different observers.

■ While a single score is not necessarily of much use in itself, observing trends over time is helpful in evaluating a patient's status.

■ Minimum ('worst') score = 3/15; maximum ('best') score = 15/15.

■ Mnemonic = 'MSE' (remember '**M**ental **S**tate **E**xamination').

Motor (best response)
6 obeys command
5 localises to pain (purposeful movement towards painful stimuli)
4 withdraws to pain
3 abnormal flexor response to pain (decelerate)
2 abnormal extensor posturing to pain (decorticate)
1 no response to pain

Speech (best verbal response)
5 orientated
4 confused conversation (sentences)
3 inappropriate speech (words)
2 incomprehensible speech (noises)
1 none

Eye opening
4 spontaneous eye opening
3 eye opening in response to vocal command
2 eye opening in response to pain
1 None

Abbreviated mental test score

■ This is a rapid assessment tool of an individual's global cognitive function (i.e. to objectively assess confused patients or to screen for signs of dementia).

■ Each correct answer = 1 point. Score ranges from 0 to 10.

■ 7–10 = grossly normal, 4–6 = impaired, 0–3 = severely impaired.

■ Low scores (e.g. <6) should warrant more detailed analysis.

Questions/tasks
1 What is your age?
2 What is the time (to nearest hour)?
3 Recall: state an address (e.g. 42 West Street), ask the patient to repeat this now, and then again at the end of the test to assess recall.
4 Ask the patient to recognise two people (e.g. yourself and a nurse).
5 What is the year?

6 What is name of the current location (e.g. hospital, patient's home)?

7 What is your date of birth?

8 Historical/factual recall, e.g. When did World War 1 start? (1915) or When did World War 2 end? (1945). Adjust this question as required.

9 What is the name of the present monarch/head of state?

10 Count from 20→1 backwards (e.g. 20, 19, 18…).

Finally, check the patient's recall of the address given in question 3.

Mini-mental state examination (MMSE)

■ Also known as the 'Folstein' test, this is more detailed than the AMTS.

■ This 30-question test assesses orientation in time and place, registration and delayed recall, attention and calculation, language skills and visual construction.

■ The MMSE has limited value in certain cases, for example in patients with frontal pathologies, acute confusion or severe dementia.

■ Performance in the test is proportional to intelligence and it should therefore not be used in isolation for diagnosis.

■ (Approximate) scores >24/30 = effectively normal, 18–23 = mild dementia, 10–17 = moderate dementia, <10 = severe dementia (the score may need to be adjusted based on educational status of the patient or, for example, if the patient is unable to complete the written parts of the test due to a physical disability).

■ Note that this test is copyrighted and, in theory, centres need to pay for permission to use the test in clinical practice.

Folstein MF, Folstein SE, McHugh PR 1975 Mini-mental state. A practical method for grading the cognitive state of patients for the clinician. J Psychiatr Res. 12(3): 189–98.

Addenbrooke's cognitive examination (ACE)

■ This is a 100-question test that assesses six aspects of cognitive function incorporates the key areas of the MMSE and includes assessment of orientation, attention, memory, language/verbal fluency and visuo-spatial ability.

■ It is more sensitive and specific than the MMSE in isolation, can detect signs of dementia at an earlier stage and can also help distinguish Alzheimer's from the other causes of dementia.

Investigating the dementias

■ Dementia is the acquired global impairment of intellect, memory and personality without impairment of consciousness.

■ There are many causes of dementia. The commonest causes are Alzheimer's disease, vascular dementia (multi-infarct) and Lewy body disease.

■ Other important causes include fronto-temporal dementia, Korsakoff's syndrome, Creutzfeldt-Jakob disease (CJD) and AIDS-related cognitive impairment.

■ Investigation should always ensure that reversible causes (which are much less common) are excluded. This requires:

• full cognitive assessment and mental state examination: ?pseuso-dementia (secondary to depression) excluded

• blood tests: full blood count, B12/folate, thyroid function (hypothyroidism); liver function tests and urea and electrolytes (?metabolic disturbance)

- imaging: CT (?subdural haematoma, tumour, abscess, hydrocephalus).

■ Further investigations such as CSF analysis, EEG or bran biopsy may be indicated if there are atypical features or the dementia is rapidly progressive.

■ A definitive diagnosis cannot be made without histological examination. This is particularly the case in patients with CJD, in which other investigations can often be normal (although EEG can show a characteristic 'periodic' pattern).

■ In practice, dementias such as Alzheimer's are diagnosed from the clinical history and assessment, which looks for characteristic neurological and neuropsychological features.

■ Neuropsychological assessment such as MMSE can be useful to monitor progression.

Epilepsy

■ A detailed history is vital, ideally from witnesses to the seizure event.

■ Accurate diagnosis is also vital, as epilepsy can have a profound impact on a patient's quality of life, affecting issues from work to driving.

■ All patients should have:

- blood tests: glucose, urea, electrolytes, calcium and LFTs (?electrolyte or metabolic disturbance)
- ECG (?cardiogenic cause)
- EEG (see below)
- MRI (?focal lesion).

■ In patients where there is diagnostic uncertainty, EEG video telemetry may be helpful

■ Toxicology screening may also be useful in certain patients.

■ EEG can have characteristic features, including:

- spike and wave: generalised large-amplitude discharges at 3–4 Hz, characteristic of absence seizures

- spike discharge: result from focal cortical damage, e.g. with partial seizures. May be bilateral, e.g. at the onset of tonic-clonic seizures

- sharp and slow wave: also results from focal abnormalities or bilaterally pre-tonic-clonic seizure

- photo convulsive discharges: occur with flash frequencies between 14 and 20 Hz, and also with other frequencies/complex pattern stimulation, particularly with children

- other patterns include: slow-wave discharges, and fast rhythms.

Remember: normal investigations *do not* exclude epilepsy (which is a clinical diagnosis).

Headaches

■ Headaches are extremely common and usually benign.

■ Red flags in headaches include:

- 'thunderclap' or sudden onset headache: investigate for SAH

- new onset headache in older patient
- consider giant cell arteritis
- ESR/CRP
- temporal artery biopsy

- headache with features of raised intracranial pressure

- worse in the morning or lying flat, on straining

- visual obscuration, papilloedema

- e.g. idiopathic intracranial hypertension, obstructive hydrocephalus, intracranial neoplasm

- if headache, neck stiffness, photophobia, fever are present, always **investigate for meningitis**.

Transient ischaemic attack (TIA) and stroke

Transient ischaemic attack (TIA)

■ TIAs are episodes of neurological dysfunction (of occlusive vascular origin) lasting less than 24 h.

■ They require urgent assessment: one-third will have a further TIA and one-third will subsequently go on have a stroke.

■ The 'ABCD2' score can predict the likelihood of subsequent stroke.

Feature	Points
Age ≥60 years	1 point
BP at presentation ≥140/90 mmHg	1 point
Clinical features:	
■ unilateral weakness	2 points
■ speech disturbance	1 point
Duration:	
■ ≥60 minutes	2 points
■ 10–59 minutes	1 point
Diabetes mellitus present	1 point

Scores and risk of subsequent stroke

■ Score 0–3: low risk.

■ Score 4–5: 6% risk of stroke in next 7 days.

■ Score 6–7: 12% risk of stroke in next 7 days.

Investigation includes

■ Blood: full blood count (?anaemia, infection), glucose (?hypoglycaemia), ESR (?vasculitis), lipid profile (?raised cholesterol).

■ Electrocardiogram (ECG): ?arrhythmia.

■ Echocardiogram: ?source of thrombo-embolus.

■ Carotid ultrasound (Doppler/duplex): ?carotid artery stenosis.

■ CT or MRI with diffusion weighting (better at identifying areas of hypoxic oedema than conventional MRI).

Stroke

■ Strokes result from the sudden loss of blood supply to an area of the brain, commonly through occlusion (thrombo-embolism) or haemorrhage of a cerebral blood vessel.

■ Stroke is a medical emergency.

■ Patients should be admitted to hospital within 3 h of symptom onset to qualify for thrombolysis treatment in cases of ischaemic stroke.

■ All patients need to have CT (or MRI) to exclude haemorrhage.

■ Thrombolytics are given if:

• symptoms/signs are consistent with a stroke

• no haemorrhage on CT/MRI

• BP < 185/100 mmHg

• platelets >100 and normal clotting

• no history of recent trauma/surgery.

■ Following emergency management, further investigations (as outlined above for TIA) may be necessary to investigate and treat the cause/risk factors for stroke.

Parkinson's disease and other movement disorders

Parkinson's disease

■ Idiopathic Parkinson's disease (IPD) is a clinical diagnosis, characterised by tremor, rigidity and bradykinesia.

■ Investigations such as MRI are not usually necessary unless additional features are present to suggest a

'Parkinsonian plus' syndrome. These features include:

- eye movement restrictions (primary feature)
- prominent autonomic features
- cerebellar signs.

■ A DaTSCAN (SPECT scanning using a radio-labelled ligand of the presynaptic dopamine amine transporter) can help differentiate IPD from essential tremor or Lewy body disease from Alzheimer's.

Other movement disorders

■ Choreas, and other involuntary movements, have many causes.

■ They frequently occur as a complication of the treatment of Parkinson's disease.

■ In other cases, exhaustive investigations may be required, taking into account the clinical features, type of movement disorder, age of onset and progression.

■ An important condition not to miss is Wilson's disease: any young adult with a movement disorder (e.g. tremor) should therefore be screened:

- serum copper (elevated) and caeruloplasmin (low) levels; urinary copper (elevated)
- slit lamp examination for Kayser-Fleischer rings.

■ Other important rare conditions include:

- Huntington's disease: requires genetic testing (following appropriate counselling)
- neuroacanthocytosis: spiky red blood cells on blood films
- Sydenham's chorea: check anti-streptolysin-O (ASO) titre and for a history of antecedent streptococcal infection.

Multiple sclerosis (MS)

■ MS is an autoimmune demyelinating disease of the CNS.

■ Clinical features play an important part in diagnosis, with objective criteria requiring two anatomically discrete demyelinating events on imaging, separated in time.

■ Note that the diagnostic criteria for MS are ever changing, and an important part of the diagnosis involves excluding other autoimmune disorders such as systemic lupus erythematosus (SLE).

■ Investigations may be performed to support the diagnosis, for example after the first demyelinating event but before a formal diagnosis can be reached. These include:

- imaging (MRI): the diagnosis of multiple sclerosis relies on imaging criteria, specifically two anatomically separate demyelinating events separated by at least 30 days. The newer MacDonald criteria (2001) allow diagnosis to be made after a single event, with the 'second' event defined as a new lesion appearing on MRI. The anatomical dissemination required (i.e. lesions at two distinct sites) can be replaced by either nine 'typical' white matter lesions on MRI or one 'enhancing' lesion (or only two 'typical' lesions if CSF studies show raised IgG or oligoclonal bands)
- CSF analysis: elevated IgG levels, presence of oligoclonal bands (proteins)
- visual and somatosensory evoked potentials (VEP, SEP) reveal delayed responses to optic nerve and sensory nerves.

Muscle disorders

■ Muscle disorders often have characteristic features which may allow diagnosis at the bedside.

■ The classical pattern is proximal limb weakness, but distal arm weakness is typical for inclusion body myositis (the commonest acquired myopathy).

■ Many muscle disorders are inherited and require specialist assessment and genetic testing.

Investigation

■ Creatine kinase (CK): elevated in the majority of patients with muscle disorders:
• can be extremely high in muscular dystrophies (e.g. Becker/Duchenne)
• CK can also be raised by denervation (e.g. MND, hypothyroidism/hypoparathyroidism, muscle trauma, seizures, drugs).

■ Nerve conduction studies/EMG:
• exclude other causes of weakness such as neuropathy
• identify myopathic or other specific changes in muscle.

■ Muscle biopsy:
• need to avoid severely affected muscles as only non-specific changes may be evident.

Acute limb and respiratory paresis

Two important causes will be considered here:
■ Guillain-Barré syndrome (GBS)
■ Myasthenia gravis (MG).

Guillain-Barré syndrome (GBS)

■ GBS is an acute polyradiculoneuropathy that affects the peripheral nerves, often following an infective trigger.

■ The diagnosis of GBS is clinical, involving a progressive weakness and sensory disturbance evolving over a 2- to 4-week period, often following an infectious episode.

■ Examination reveals varying degrees of limb weakness, absent reflexes, and sensory disturbance.

Investigation

■ Patients may have autonomic instability and it is important to monitor blood pressure and ECG.

■ Measurement of vital capacity is important in detecting one of the most severe complications of GBS – respiratory paralysis.

■ Lumbar puncture: CSF can show an elevated protein level without an increased cell count

■ Neurophysiology: EMG/nerve conduction studies can show prolonged distal latencies, slowed conduction and conduction block.

Note that many of the tests (e.g. CSF analysis and nerve conduction studies) can often be normal during the first few days of the illness).

Myasthenia gravis (MG)

■ MG is a disorder that affects the neuromuscular junction (NMJ). It may present acutely with limb, facial, extra-ocular, bulbar and respiratory weakness.

■ The weakness is fatigable, with no sensory symptoms or signs. Pupil reflexes remain intact (cf. botulism).

Investigation

The diagnosis of MG is based on clinical features but helpful investigations include the following.

■ Forced vital capacity (FVC): as for GBS, there is a risk of respiratory muscle paralysis, hence an important investigation is FVC, which may be supplemented with an arterial blood gas (ABG) to ensure adequate perfusion.

■ Acetylcholine receptor antibody: these are present in most (>85%) cases of myasthenia gravis. They are markers of severity or treatment response.

■ Anti-MuSK antibodies: these can be detected in a small proportion of cases of MG (<10%). About 50% of acetylcholine receptor seronegative patients show anti-MuSK positivity – often those with prominent facial, bulbar and respiratory muscle involvement.

■ Tensilon (edrophonium) test:
• this is a short acting anticholinesterase that can be used to help diagnose MG
• following a test dose of 2 mg IV (to check for sensitivity), a larger (8 mg) dose of Tensilon is administered. This should improve muscle strength and reduce fatigability for a brief period (approximately 1 min). Atropine may be required to reverse associated autonomic side-effects (e.g. sweating, dizziness).

■ Single fibre EMG: can show a 'jitter and block' pattern

■ CT chest: to identify thymoma (a tumour associated with MG).

Chapter 8
HAEMATOLOGY

Introduction

This chapter will consider several aspects of one of the most commonly used investigations: the blood test. In particular, consideration will be given to the different lineages encompassed by the full blood count. The causes and investigation of abnormalities such as anaemias, deranged clotting function and infection will be discussed, as these are common tests encountered both in medical examinations and clinical practice. Finally, we will look at some of the drugs that affect coagulation and will consider the basics of blood transfusion and some commonly used inflammatory markers.

Topics covered
- Components of the full blood count
- Haematinics
- Anaemia
- Haemolytic anaemia
- Pancytopaenia and myeloproliferative disorders

- Blood films
- Coagulopathy (bleeding disorders)
- Anticoagulant/antiplatelet/thrombolytic agents
- Myeloproliferative disorders
- Blood transfusion
- Inflammatory markers

Components of the full blood count

Haemoglobin (Hb)

> *Normal range:* 13–18 g/dL (males), 11.5–16 g/dL (females)

Increased haemoglobin (polycythaemia)
Causes: primary
- Polycythaemia rubra vera (PRV, rare).

Relative
- On the wards: most commonly due to dehydration.
- Burns (also secondary due to dehydration).

Causes: secondary
- Hypoxia:
- consequence of chronic obstructive pulmonary disease (COPD)
- living at high altitude
- smoking.
- Erythropoietin (epo) use.
See 'Packed cell volume/haematocrit' section below.

The hands-on guide to data interpretation. By S. Abraham, K. Kulkarni, R. Madhu and D. Provan. Published 2010 by Blackwell Publishing Ltd.

Further investigation of polycythaemia

As there are a number of causes of polycythaemia, further investigations can be helpful in distinguishing the root cause.

■ Oxygen saturations/ABG – ? hypoxia.

■ Renal function and erythropoietin levels – ?renal failure/epo use ?polycystic kidney disease.

■ Liver/spleen assessment (e.g. liver function tests, abdomen imaging) – ? malignancy.

■ JAK2 gene mutation analysis (diagnostic test for PRV).

■ Further abdominal imaging – ?malignancy.

Decreased haemoglobin (anaemia)

■ Anaemia = Hb below the expected level for age and gender.

■ Not a stand-alone diagnosis: always look for an underlying cause.

■ There are many potential causes.

■ The main parameter used to classify anaemia is the mean corpuscular volume (MCV). This is a measure of the volume of the red blood cells (RBCs).

Further investigation of anaemia

■ Further blood investigations – ?haematological cause ?nutritional deficiency ?renal cause ?haemolysis:

• mean corpuscular volume (MCV)
• packed cell volume (PCV)/haematocrit (Hct)
• blood film
• haematinics (B12, folate, iron studies)
• renal function
• liver function.

■ Gastrointestinal (GI) investigation – ?blood loss:

• upper GI tract endoscopy (oesophagealgastroduodenoscopy, OGD)
• lower GI tract endoscopy (rigid/flexible sigmoidoscopy, colonoscopy)
• barium studies
• imaging (CT colonoscopy).

Mean corpuscular volume (MCV)

Normal range: 76–96 fL

■ This is a measure of average RBC volume.

■ MCV >96 fL = **macrocytic (higher volume RBCs)**.

■ MCV <76 fL = **microcytic (lower volume RBCs)**.

■ MCV 76–96 fL = **normocytic**.

NB: If causes of both, macrocytosis and microcytosis are present, it is possible to have a combined picture (with a resultant 'normocytic' MCV).

Mean cell haemoglobin (MCH)/mean cell haemoglobin concentration (MCHC)

■ These are further measures that can be used to investigate anaemias.

■ For example, a low MCH and MCHC are typical of hypochromic anaemias.

■ MCH = estimation of the Hb in an average erythrocyte.

■ MCHC = estimated mean Hb concentration in a given volume of cells.

Normal ranges: MCH = 27–32 pg/cell; MCHC = 31–35 g/dL.

Packed cell volume (PCV)/haematocrit (Hct)

This is a measure of the proportion (percentage) of the blood volume occupied by RBCs.

> *Normal range (Hct):* 40–50% (males), 36–45% (females)

Increased
- Dehydration (decreased plasma volume)
- Polycythaemia (raised red cell mass) – number of causes

Decreased
- Anaemia
- Haemorrhage
- Bone marrow failure
- Over-hydration
- Rheumatoid arthritis (anaemia of chronic disease)

White cell count (WCC)

- The differential WCC is part of the full blood count (FBC).
- Raised levels of particular cell lines can help determine the aetiology of the disease process (e.g. bacterial versus viral origin).

> *Normal range:* 4–11 × 10^9/L (total WCC)

Neutrophils
- These are the most abundant type of white blood cell (WBC).
- Their presence is associated with a range of causes.

> *Normal range:* 2.5–7.5 × 10^9/L (usually accounts for 40–75% of WCC)

Increased
- Bacterial infection
- Trauma: surgery, burns, post myocardial infarction, haemorrhage
- Inflammation
- Polymyalgia
- Myeloproliferative disorders (especially myeloid leukaemia)
- Drugs (e.g. steroids)
- Disseminated malignancy

Decreased
- Viral infections
- Drugs (e.g. carbimazole, sulfonamides, clozapine)
- Hypersplenism
- Anti-neutrophil antibodies (e.g. autoimmune phenomenon in systemic lupus erythematosus or rheumatoid arthritis – also Felty's syndrome)
- Increased destruction
- Bone marrow failure (i.e. decreased production) – can be post-chemotherapy/radiotherapy

Lymphocytes

> *Normal range:* 1.5–4.0 × 10^9/L (usually account for 20–45% of WCC)

Increased
- Viral infection
- Chronic lymphocytic leukaemia

Decreased
- Steroid therapy
- SLE

- Marrow infiltration
- Post chemotherapy/radiotherapy

Monocytes

> *Normal range:* 0.2–0.8 × 10⁹/L (usually account for 2–10% of WCC)

Increased
- Acute and chronic infection (e.g. tuberculosis, protozoal)
- Malignancy

Decreased
- Bone marrow failure

Eosinophils

> *Normal range:* 0.04–0.44 × 10⁹/L (usually account for 1–6% of WCC)

Increased
- Asthma/eczema (and other atopic/ allergic conditions)
- Parasitic infections (e.g. hookworm, hydatid)
- Urticaria
- Polyarteritis nodosa (PAN)
- Malignancy (e.g. lymphoma)
- Aspergillosis (allergic bronchopulmonary)
- Adrenal insufficiency

Decreased
- Bone marrow failure

Basophils

> *Normal range:* 0.0–0.1 × 109/L (usually account for 0–1% of WCC)

Increased
- Viral infection
- Urticaria
- Myxoedema (hypothyroidism)
- Haemolysis
- Malignant disease
- PRV

Decreased
Difficult to demonstrate (due to very low 'normal' count).

Platelets

> *Normal range:* 150–400 × 10⁹/L

- A low platelet count (thrombocytopaenia) can lead to haemorrhage due to impaired coagulation.
- Symptoms/signs are rare with platelet counts >50 × 10⁹/L.
- A persistently high platelet count (thrombocytosis) can lead to an increased risk of venous and arterial thrombotic events.

Increased (thrombocytosis)
Primary
- Essential thrombocythaemia
- Myelodysplasia

Secondary (reactive)
- Trauma (e.g. post-surgery)
- Active bleeding
- Infection
- Post-splenectomy
- Malignancy (e.g. Hodgkin's disease, chronic myeloid leukaemia)
- Pregnancy
- Inflammation (e.g. chronic inflammatory diseases such as rheumatoid arthritis or Crohn's disease)

Decreased (thrombocytopaenia)

Impaired platelet production

■ Marrow failure – can be due to any of the causes of pancytopaenia, e.g. leukaemia, myelofibrosis, megaloblastic anaemia, aplastic anaemia, drugs such as hydroxyurea, etc.

Increased platelet destruction

■ Autoimmune, DIC, massive transfusion, thrombotic thrombocytopaenic purpura (TTP), hypersplenism, haemolytic uraemic syndrome (HUS, e.g. with *E. coli* 0157 infection).

Haematinics

■ These studies include measurement of the levels of iron, vitamin B12 and folate.

■ Absorption of the elements takes place at the following locations:</BL

- iron: duodenum, jejunum
- B12: terminal ileum
- folate: small bowel.

Iron

■ Absorbed in the ferrous (Fe^{2+}) state.

■ Stored as ferritin and haemosiderin.

■ Ferritin is also an acute-phase protein (like CRP, see below).

■ Red cells transport iron via transferrin receptors.

■ Soluble transferrin receptors are an accurate marker of body iron stores.

In iron deficiency

■ Anaemia: microcytic.

■ Serum iron: low.

■ Ferritin: low.

■ Transferrin: increased (greater numbers of receptors).

■ Total iron binding capacity (TIBC): increased (lots of free binding sites).

B12

Causes of deficiency

■ Dietary (e.g. vegan diet).

■ Impaired absorption:

- pernicious anaemia (autoimmune condition – antibodies against gastric parietal cells leading to impaired intrinsic factor production, which is required for B12 absorption)
- gastrectomy
- bacterial overgrowth
- tropical sprue
- ileal disease (Crohn's, resection)
- fish tapeworm.

■ Abnormal metabolism: congenital transcobalamin deficiency (very rare).

Schilling test

This can be used to help determine the cause of the B12 deficiency.

■ Two doses of vitamin B12 are given. One is radio-labelled and given orally. The other dose is given intramuscularly.

■ Urine is collected over 24h.

■ In normal people, a proportion of the oral B12 is absorbed and more than 10% of this excreted in the urine.

■ In B12 malabsorption, less than this is excreted in the urine.

■ The test is then repeated with oral intrinsic factor being administered with the oral dose of B12.

■ If the results are normal, then the cause of B12 deficiency is likely to be due to pernicious anaemia (lack of intrinsic factor). If the test is still abnormal, the problem is likely to be impaired ileal absorption.

Folate

Causes of deficiency

■ Dietary
• Deficiency or malabsorption
• Alcohol excess
• Gastrointestinal disease: coeliac disease, Crohn's disease
■ Iatrogenic
• Drugs: phenytoin, methotrexate, trimethoprim
• Gastrectomy, bowel resection
■ Increased use of folate
• Pregnancy and lactation
• Malignancy
• Inflammatory disease

NB: A mixed state of microcytosis and macrocytosis (for example, due to combined iron and vitamin B12 deficiency in malabsorptive states) can lead to an overall picture of a normocytic anaemia (with a dimorphic population of cells).

Anaemia

Causes

Microcytic
■ Iron deficiency
■ Thalassaemia
■ Long-standing anaemia of chronic disease
■ Congenital sideroblastic anaemia (very rare)

Normocytic
■ Anaemia of chronic disease
■ Bone marrow failure
■ Renal failure
■ Hypothyroidism (also macrocytic)
■ Pregnancy (may be spurious result due to increase in plasma volume)

Macrocytic
Megaloblastic
■ B12 or folate deficiency (can also be seen in those who abuse alcohol)
■ Anti-folate drugs (e.g. phenytoin)

Normoblastic
■ Alcohol excess
■ Liver disease
■ Reticulocytosis
■ Cytotoxic drugs (e.g. hydroxyurea, azathioprine)
■ Marrow infiltration
■ Haemolysis (usually macrocytic)
■ Hypothyroidism
■ Pregnancy
■ Myelodysplasia

NB: 'Megaloblastic' means that there are features of nuclear:cytoplasmic asynchrony. With B12/folate assays being easier and cheaper to perform than in the past, bone marrow biopsies (necessary to determine normoblastic versus megaloblastic) are less commonly performed.

Haemolytic anaemia

■ This type of anaemia is caused by an abnormally increased destruction of RBCs.
■ It is important to note that haemolysis in itself does not always lead to clinically detectable anaemia – there is capacity for a large compensatory increase in the production of erythroid stem cells as well as increases in the bone marrow volume.

Investigation
■ Increased number of reticulocytes (immature red blood cells) and RBC fragments (schistocytes) on a peripheral blood film

- Low haptoglobin concentration
- Elevated lactate dehydrogenase (LDH)
- Elevated unconjugated bilirubin
- Positive direct Coombs' test (autoimmune haemolysis)
- Osmotic fragility test (hereditary spherocytosis)
- Haemosiderin and urobilinogen in the urine (suggests chronic intravascular haemolysis)

Causes of reticulocytosis
- Haemolysis
- Haemorrhage
- Marrow infiltration (for example, secondary to malignancy)

Causes of haemolytic anaemia

These can be divided into two groups.

Congenital (genetic basis)
- Haemoglobin abnormalities – thalassaemia, sickle cell disease.
- Red cell membrane abnormalities – hereditary spherocytosis.
- Metabolic defects – glucose-6-phosphate dehydrogenase deficiency (G6PD), pyruvate kinase deficiency (PKD).

Acquired
- Autoimmune. Can be 'warm' or 'cold' (depending on the temperature at which antibodies bind to red cells).
- Warm antibody mediated: commonest. Often idiopathic, drug related (e.g. penicillin/cephalosporins) or associated with connective tissue disorders such as systemic lupus erythematosus. Usually IgG mediated.

- Cold antibody mediated: again, often idiopathic, or secondary to underlying conditions such as lympho-proliferative disease (e.g. lymphoma) or infection (e.g. infectious mononucleosis – EBV, HIV or *Mycoplasma* pneumonia – usually IgM).
- Alloimmune – haemolytic transfusion reactions, haemolytic disease of the newborn.
- Drug induced (e.g. penicillin).
- Non-immune – trauma, mechanical (prosthetic heart valves, March haemoglobinuria), secondary to systemic disease.

Antiglobulin (Coombs') test

Direct
- This is used in the detection of autoimmune haemolytic anaemias.
- Anti-human globulin (Coombs' reagent) is added to a sample of the patient's red cells.
- If the patient's red cells are coated (sensitised) with auto-antibodies, then agglutination occurs: a positive test.

Indirect
- This is used in pre-blood transfusion testing ('cross matching'), or in the pre-natal testing of pregnant women.
- The purpose is to detect unbound serum anti-red cell antibodies.
- Serum (extracted from the patient's blood) is added to red cells of a known antigenicity.
- If agglutination occurs, the test is positive.

Osmotic fragility tests

- Used to determine the degree of red cell rupture when exposed to saline at varying concentrations.

■ Patient red cells are placed into a solution of saline (of varying concentration).

■ The aim is to try to see how much water the cells can take up before they burst.

■ The result reflects the shape of the red cell, i.e. spherical red cells (spherocytes) can only take up small amount of fluid before rupturing whereas a normal disc-shaped red cell can avoid rupture due to its ability to take up more fluid before rupture occurs. A positive test therefore suggests a condition such as hereditary spherocytosis.

Pancytopaenia

Pancytopaenia is a global lack of cells in the blood (low RBC, WBC and platelet counts).

Causes

■ Bone marrow failure
• Aplastic anaemia (pancytopaenia with no leukaemic, cancerous or abnormal cells in the blood) (see below)
• Myelodysplasia
• Malignancy (acute leukaemia, lymphoma, myeloma, metastases, myelofibrosis) or its treatment (e.g. chemotherapy)
• HIV
■ Paroxysmal nocturnal haemoglobinuria
■ Infections (e.g. disseminated tuberculosis, Leishmaniasis)
■ Severe folate/B12 deficiency (e.g. secondary to pernicious anaemia)
■ Drugs
■ Hypersplenism

Further investigation

■ Blood: FBC, blood film, haematinics, renal/liver function, thyroid function.
■ Imaging: as appropriate, if malignancy suspected,
■ Invasive: bone marrow biopsy.

Aplastic anaemia

■ This is a state where the bone marrow fails to produce sufficient precursor cells.
■ Signs/symptoms reflect the lack of each blood-cell lineage:
• anaemia → fatigue, shortness of breath, pallor (low RBC)
• leucopaenia → infection (low WBC)
• thrombocytopaenia → haemorrhage (low platelets).

Causes

■ Congenital
• Fanconi's
■ Acquired
• Autoimmune
• Chemicals (e.g. benzene, insecticides)
• Drugs (e.g. chemotherapeutic agents, chloramphenicol, carbamazepine, phenytoin, phenylbutazone)
• Radiation
• Infection: viral (e.g. hepatitis, HIV) or non-viral (e.g. tuberculosis)

Blood films

Abnormally shaped red blood cells or pathological red blood cells can be characteristic of various pathologies.

Red blood cell abnormalities

Anisocytosis	Red cells of varying size, e.g. megaloblastic anaemia, thalassaemia
Auer rods	Needle-like clumps of granular material seen in acute myeloid leukaemia (AML)
Basophilic stripping	Lead poisoning, thalassaemia
Blasts	Precursor cells, e.g. leukaemias and myelofibrosis
Burr cell (echinocyte)	Spherical RBC with projections or 'spicules', e.g. microangiopathic haemolytic anaemia, uraemia, pyruvate kinase deficiency
Elliptocytes	Oval/elongated RCB with central pallor, e.g. hereditary elliptocytosis
Heinz bodies	Denatured round Hb inclusions within RBCs – bite cells, e.g. alpha-thalassaemia, G6PD and oxidant-drug use
Howell-Jolly bodies	Nuclear remnants, e.g. post-splenectomy
Hypochromia	Decreased density colour of red blood cells, e.g. iron deficiency anaemias, thalassaemia, sideroblastic anaemia
Normoblasts	Immature red cells, e.g. leucoerythoblastic anaemias, haemolysis
Pappenheimer bodies	Iron containing granules, e.g. post-splenectomy, haemolytic anaemias, sideroblastic anaemias, lead poisoning
Pencil cells	Similar to elliptocyte, e.g. iron deficiency
Poikilocytes	Iron deficiency, myelofibrosis, thalassaemia
Rouleaux formation	Stacked red cells, the equivalent of raised ESR, e.g. in myeloma
Schistocyte	Fragmented RCB, e.g. haemolytic anaemia, disseminated intravascular coagulation (DIC), uraemia, severe burns
Sickle cells	E.g. sickle cell
Spherocytes	E.g. hereditary spherocytosis
Spurr cell (acanthocyte)	Irregular thorny appearance, e.g. post-splenectomy, liver disease, disseminated intravascular coagulation (DIC)
Target cell	Increased surface area-volume ratio (bull's-eye appearance), e.g. thalassaemia, post-splenectomy, iron deficiency, liver disease

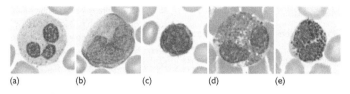

Figure 8.1: (a) Neutrophil, (b) monocyte, (c) lymphocyte, (d) eosinophil and (e) basophil

Coagulopathy (bleeding disorders)

Coagulation cascade

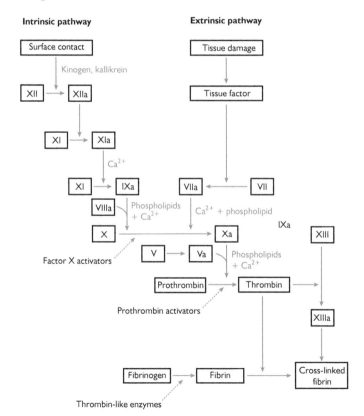

Figure 8.2: Coagulation cascade

Haemostasis

Stopping bleeding once it has started (haemostasis) is a complicated process relying on many factors coming together in the appropriate order.

1 Vessel wall constriction
2 Platelet activation
3 Activation of the clotting cascade
Bleeding disorders usually mean a defect in any of these three components.

Coagulopathy

This is impaired clotting.

Investigation
■ FBC and blood film
■ Bleeding time (deranged in von Willebrand's disease and also with anti-platelet agents, e.g. aspirin)
■ Coagulation tests

Coagulation tests
Prothrombin time (PT)
■ Measure of the 'extrinsic' system.
■ Can also be expressed as a ratio to the 'normal' PT ($\approx$12–15 s +/– individual laboratory compensation), known as international normalised ratio (INR).
■ As PT can vary depending on the laboratory assay used, this is of benefit when comparing results across centres, for example when monitoring warfarin therapy and also in detecting any abnormality of factors I, II, V, VII and X.
■ Warfarin increases the INR.

Activated partial thromboplastin time (APTT)
■ Measure of the 'intrinsic' system.
■ The normal time is $\approx$40–50 s, but is prolonged with factor I, II, V, VIII, IX, XI, XII (note *not* factor VII).

■ Heparin therapy increases the APTT (used for monitoring). Note that low-molecular weight heparins cannot be properly monitored using the APTT *(see below)*.

Thrombin time (TT)
■ Usually prolonged with fibrinogen deficiency, DIC or with heparin/fibrin degradation product (FDP) use.

Specific tests (e.g. individual factor assays)
Haematology specialist should be consulted. Examples include the following.
■ Factor Xa assay is used to check the effects of low molecular weight heparin (LMWH) therapy.
■ Factor VIII/IX levels in haemophilia.

Fibrin degradation products (D-dimer)
■ Levels increased by fibrinolysis (e.g. in DIC or venous thrombo-embolism, such as deep-venous thrombosis, DVT).
■ When investigating DVT remember to consider the fact that elevated d-dimer values are not only caused by DVT.

DIC

■ This is a 'consumptive coagulopathy', i.e. a process of spontaneous intravascular coagulation.
■ As well as an increased risk of thrombosis, there is paradoxically also an increased risk of haemorrhage.
■ There are many causes. These include:
• sepsis/critically ill patient (e.g. meningococcal, malarial)
• malignancy
• obstetric (e.g. eclampsia, placental abruption/praevia, amniotic fluid embolus)
• blood transfusion reaction (e.g. incompatibility)
• liver disease (e.g. cirrhosis).

Investigation
- Deranged clotting function
- Elevated PT/APTT
- Elevated d-dimer
- Low fibrinogen
- Low platelets (high consumption)

Anticoagulant/antiplatelet/thrombolytic agents

Drug	Mechanism of action
Antiplatelet	
Aspirin	Cyclooxygenase (COX) inhibition
Clopidogrel/Ticlopidine	Adenosine diphosphate (ADP) receptor inhibitors
Cilostazol	Phosphodiesterase inhibitor
Abciximab, Tirofiban, etc.	Glycoprotein IIb/IIIa inhibitors (e.g. IV use in acute myocardial infarction)
Dipyridamole	Adenosine re-uptake inhibitor
Anticoagulant	
Heparin	Activates anti-thrombin III (monitor with APTT)
Low-molecular weight heparin (LMWH)	Factor Xa inhibitor (can measure anti-Xa activity in certain scenarios, e.g. pregnant women with venous thromboembolism with very low/high body weights – not otherwise routinely measured
Warfarin	Vitamin K antagonist (monitor with INR)
Fondaparinux	Synthetic factor Xa inhibitor
Thrombolytic	
Recombinant tissue-plasminogen activator (rt-PA), reteplase, etc.	
Streptokinase, urokinase, etc.	Fibrin degradation

Anticoagulation during pregnancy

- Pregnancy is a risk factor for venous thromboembolism (VTE).
- Women with a previous VTE or at risk for VTE should receive antenatal thromboprophylaxis with LMWH.
- Oral anticoagulants (e.g. warfarin) are associated with the development of congenital abnormalities so should be avoided during pregnancy.

Myeloproliferative disorders

These involve the uncontrolled proliferation of a particular cell line, usually the myeloid, erythroid or megakaryocyte lineage. They include the following.

■ Myeloid leukaemia (WBC proliferation)

■ Essential thrombocythaemia (platelet proliferation)

■ Polycythaemia rubra vera (RBC proliferation)

■ Myelofibrosis (replacement of marrow architecture with fibrous connective tissue)

Investigation

■ Blood count and film

■ Bone marrow aspirate and trephine biopsy

■ Other investigations include genetic studies, e.g. JAK 2 mutation for myelofibrosis, or blood/marrow cytogenetics for Philadelphia chromosome – t(9;22)

Having one of these conditions can predispose to the others, so they should not be considered in isolation.

Blood transfusion

■ Blood groups are determined by antigens on the surface of RBCs.

■ Although only the ABO and Rh blood groups will be considered here, at least 400 blood group systems have been identified (such as the Kell and Duffy systems).

■ Incompatibility of any of these groups may cause transfusion reactions, to varying degrees of severity.

The ABO system

Phenotype	Genotype	Antigens	Antibodies
O	OO	None	Anti-A; Anti-B
A	AO: AA	A	Anti-B
B	BO: BB	B	Anti-A
AB	AB	A and B	None

■ Incompatibility with Rh groups causes problems, particularly for the newborn.

■ For example, if the mother is Rh(D) negative and the foetus is Rh(D) positive, the mother will make IgG antibodies against Rh(D). This leads to haemolysis of foetal red cells (haemolytic disease of the newborn).

■ Generally, mothers are given prophylaxis against this by using intramuscular anti-D antibody during pregnancy; the prophylactic anti-D prevents sensitisation after the red cells reach the mother's circulation.

Inflammatory markers

■ Erythrocyte sedimentation rate (ESR) and C-reactive protein (CRP) are often used in clinical practice as general markers of inflammation.

■ Other markers include haptoglobulins, ferritin and α-1-antitrypsin, although there are many more.

■ Markers reflect levels of the inflammatory mediators in the blood. There is often a concomitant fall in serum albumin at times of inflammation due to increased permeability of the capillaries and release of albumin into the extravascular space.

Erythrocyte sedimentation rate (ESR)

■ This is the rate of fall of RBCs in a column of anti-coagulated blood.

■ A raised ESR indicates the presence of certain proteins in the blood, such as fibrinogen.

■ These proteins tend to make the column of red cells fall more quickly. It is a non-specific indicator of the presence of disease and a measure of acute phase response.

■ Usually two raised ESR readings are taken before any medical intervention occurs unless the ESR is very high.

■ ESR is often used to monitor the progress of chronic inflammatory conditions such as rheumatoid arthritis and systemic vasculitides.

Increased
■ Age
■ Female
■ Inflammation
■ Anaemia

Decreased
■ Often due to a spurious sample
■ Sickle cell disease

■ Polycythaemia rubra vera (due to high red cell concentration)
■ Cryoglobulinaemia

Westergren method for determining ESR
■ Men: age in years/2
■ Women: (age in years + 10)/2

Normal range: <20 mm/h (average)

C-reactive protein (CRP)

■ This is another acute phase protein (a pentraxin).

■ It is also produced in acute phase of inflammation, synthesised in the liver within hours of an inflammatory event and falls over 2–3 days, binding strongly to phospholipids.

■ It reflects clinical condition of patient more quickly than the ESR, but less useful for monitoring chronic conditions than ESR.

Conditions where CRP monitoring may be useful
■ Following major surgery
■ (Bacterial) infection
■ When a general indicator of sepsis is needed

Normal range: 0–6 mg/L

Chapter 9
RHEUMATOLOGY

Introduction

Broadly speaking, rheumatology can be divided into the inflammatory arthropathies, connective tissue diseases and mechanical musculoskeletal disorders. History and examination will often reveal clues as to the nature and severity of the presenting condition, as many of these disorders exhibit characteristic patterns of symptoms and signs. Common presentations include pain, stiffness and deformity – symptoms common to a number of rheumatological disorders. A few 'red flag' features can suggest more serious or acute underlying pathology, for example systemic illness, headache, single joint involvement or neurological symptoms. Further investigation, usually in the form of analysis of blood/aspirate samples or imaging can prove a useful diagnostic adjunct. This section aims to provide an overview of some of the investigative tools for rheumatological disease.

Topics covered
- Basic investigations
- Rheumatoid factor
- Seronegative spondyloarthritis
- Other plasma auto-antibodies associated with disease
- Ophthalmic manifestations of systemic disease
- Human leucocyte antigen (HLA) system
- Synovial fluid analysis
- X-ray changes in rheumatological disease

Basic investigations

The investigations outlined below are of use both in the initial investigation of a condition and in monitoring response to treatment. For example, the inflammatory marker ESR can be used in monitoring treatment response in conditions such as temporal arteritis or rheumatoid arthritis.

Blood

- Full blood count (?anaemia of chronic disease, ?deficiencies, Hb monitoring when using marrow-toxic drugs or gold/penicillamine, etc., ?bleeding secondary to non-steroidal anti-inflammatory drug (NSAID) use).
- C-reactive protein (CRP): acute phase plasma protein (non-specific marker of inflammation).
- Erythrocyte sedimentation rate (ESR) (non-specific marker of inflammatory disease activity).

The hands-on guide to data interpretation. By S. Abraham, K. Kulkarni, R. Madhu and D. Provan.
Published 2010 by Blackwell Publishing Ltd.

- Urea and electrolytes (?renal damage as part of a systemic connective tissue disease or secondary to NSAID use).
- Liver function tests (?drug toxicity, ?raised alkaline phosphatase – non-specific marker of bony disease).
- Uric acid (?gout – although this is not always raised in acute disease).
- Infective markers (e.g. bacterial culture, viral serology/titres – rheumatological disease can often have an infection-triggered aetiology).
- Specific markers (e.g. parathyroid hormone, other electrolytes such as calcium, specific immune markers such as autoantibodies (e.g. rheumatoid factor), genetic markers (e.g. HLA type)).
- Serology: (? positive viral serology).

Histology/Microbiology

- Culture and microscopy (e.g. of joint effusion aspirates – send for infective cultures as well as microscopy for crystals).
- Biopsy (e.g. of skin, synovium, blood vessel, muscle, etc.): can be used to examine tissue for the presence of inflammatory cells (e.g. temporal artery biopsy in suspected temporal arteritis).

Imaging/invasive

- Arthroscopy: allows direct visualisation of joints; can also be therapeutic, e.g. by aspiration of effusions.
- X-ray: while of limited value for soft tissue inflammation, X-rays may demonstrate bony abnormalities as well as other pathologies (e.g. malignancy on chest X-ray).
- Ultrasound: this can be used to visualise mass lesions (e.g. cysts) or vascular pathology.

- MRI/CT: magnetic resonance imaging is particularly good for imaging soft tissues, whereas computed tomography provides good imaging of bony lesions.

Rheumatoid factor (RF)

- This is an IgM autoantibody against the Fc portion of IgG. It is positive in approximately 75% of patients with rheumatoid arthritis.
- It is not diagnostic of rheumatoid arthritis since it may be increased in many other disease processes. However, the higher the level of rheumatoid factor early on in rheumatoid arthritis, the worse the disease process (prognosis) is likely to be.

Diseases in which RF is increased

- Rheumatoid arthritis

Other rheumatic diseases
- Sjögren's syndrome
- Felty's syndrome (RA + moderate splenomegaly + neutropaenia)
- Systemic sclerosis
- Systemic lupus erythematosus
- Polymyositis/dermatomyositis
- Juvenile arthropathy

Infection
Viral
- Hepatitis
- Infectious mononucleosis

Bacterial
- *Mycobacterium tuberculosis*
- Leprosy

- Endocarditis
- Syphilis

Other
- Sarcoidosis
- Cryoglobulinaemia

'Normal' individuals
- Up to 10% of the population, especially in the elderly.

Seronegative spondyloarthritis

■ These are a range of arthritides associated with the absence of rheumatoid factor positivity.

■ They may have an association with human leucocyte antigen (HLA) B-27.

■ Common features of these conditions include the presence of sacroiliitis (sacroiliac joint inflammation) and spondylitis (vertebral inflammation).

■ X-ray imaging can be of use to visualise general changes such as sacroiliitis or more specific changes (e.g. fusion of lumbar vertebral bodies and calcification of annulus fibrosis/interspinous segments in ankylosing spondylitis).

■ These conditions include:
- ankylosing spondylitis
- Reiter's syndrome
- psoriatic arthropathy
- enteropathic arthropathy (associated with inflammatory bowel disease)
- Behçet's syndrome.

Other plasma autoantibodies associated with disease

Plasma autoantibody	Disease	%
Antinuclear antibody (ANA)	Autoimmune hepatitis	100
	Systemic lupus erythematosus (SLE)	95
	Systemic sclerosis	95
	Sjögren's syndrome	75
	Myasthenia gravis	50
	Rheumatoid arthritis	30
	Juvenile idiopathic arthritis	30
	'Normal' individuals	up to 10
Anti-smooth muscle antibodies (ASMA)	Chronic active hepatitis	Up to 90
	Primary biliary cirrhosis	Up to 70
	Viral infection	Up to 40
	'Normal' individuals	Up to 10
Anti-Ro	SLE	40–50
	Sjögren's syndrome	60–70
Anti-La	Sjögren's syndrome	25–50
	SLE	5–10
Anti Jo-1	Polymyositis	18–20
	Dermatomyositis	2–5

(Continued)

(Continued)

Plasma autoantibody	Disease	%
Antiphospholipid antibodies	Antiphospholipid syndrome	80–90
	SLE	20–30
Anti-Topo I [scl70] antibodies	Diffuse cutaneous systemic sclerosis	60–70
Anti-centromere antibodies	Limited cutaneous systemic sclerosis (CREST syndrome)	80–90
Anti-double-stranded DNA (anti-dsDNA) antibodies	SLE	60 (in active disease)
Anti-neutrophil cytoplasmic antibodies (ANCA):		
1. cANCA (classical)	Wegener's granulomatosis	>90
2. pANCA (perinuclear)	Microscopic polyarteritis NB: Both ANCA types may be raised in Churg-Strauss syndrome (asthma + eosinophilic vasculitis + rhinitis + sinusitis)	75
Reticulin antibodies	Coeliac disease	35
	Crohn's disease	25
	Dermatitis herpetiformis	20
	'Normal' individuals	<5
Anti-mitochondrial antibody	Primary biliary cirrhosis	>60
	Idiopathic cirrhosis	25
	'Normal' individuals	<1

Anti-cyclic citrullinated peptide (anti-CCP) antibodies

■ These are potentially important surrogate markers for diagnosis and prognosis in rheumatoid arthritis (RA).
■ They are as sensitive as and more specific (specificity 95–98%) than IgM rheumatoid factors (RF) in early and fully established disease.
■ Anti-CCP may be detected in healthy individuals years before onset of clinical RA, and can be used to predict the development of erosive RA, as well as RA from undifferentiated arthritis.
■ They may be detected in roughly 50% of patients with early RA (e.g. after 3–6 months of symptoms).

Complement (C3 and C4)

■ The complement system is one of the natural defence mechanisms that protect the human body from infections and perhaps tumours.
■ Complement testing may be indicated in cases of recurrent infection or inflammation/angioedema. It can also be helpful in monitoring the activity of autoimmune diseases such as systemic lupus erythematosus (SLE) and immune complex-related diseases (e.g. glomerulonephritis and vasculitis).
■ While C3 and C4 levels are usually measured in the first instance, other components of the complement cascade can also be measured (e.g. C1 esterase

inhibitor (functional activity and concentration for hereditary angio-oedema or total complement activity – CH50/CH100)).

Decreased complement levels
■ Recurrent infections (usually bacterial)
■ Autoimmune diseases (including SLE and vasculitis)
■ Hereditary/acquired angioedema (specifically c1 esterase inhibitor)
■ Renal disease (including glomerulonephritis, lupus nephritis, membranous nephritis, IgA nephropathy)
■ Malnutrition

■ Septicaemia
■ Immune complex diseases

Increased complement levels
■ Acute or chronic inflammation (with other acute phase proteins)

Ophthalmic manifestations of systemic disease

A number of systemic and autoimmune diseases have ophthalmic manifestations.

Condition	Symptoms	Associated disease
Uveitis	Blurring of vision; eye redness; ocular pain; photophobia	Ankylosing spondylitis (25%) Juvenile idiopathic arthropathy Behçet's disease Reiter's disease (rare) Psoriatic arthropathy *Other* Syphilis Tuberculosis (TB) Leprosy Crohn's disease Ulcerative colitis Sarcoidosis
Conjunctivitis	Soreness; grittiness; redness; discharge	Reiter's disease (triad of urethritis, conjunctivitis and oligoarthritis) Psoriatic arthropathy
Episcleritis	Mild sectoral redness; no/mild discomfort; rare association with systemic disease	Rheumatoid arthritis Polyarteritis nodosa Systemic lupus erythematosus (SLE)
Scleritis	Redness; intense pain;	Rheumatoid arthritis Wegener's
Keratoconjunctiva sicca	Grittiness; burning; photophobia; lid heaviness; ocular fatigue	Rheumatoid arthritis Primary Sjögren's syndrome SLE
Orbital oedema		Dermatomyositis

Schirmer's test

Dry eyes (keratoconjunctivitis sicca) can occur alone or in combination with a systemic disorder (Sjögren's syndrome). Schirmer's test can be employed to determine whether normal tear production is present or not. Other causes of dry eyes include increasing age (especially perimenopausal and postmenopausal women), blepharitis, exposure and drugs (anticholinergics).

Protocol
- Filter paper placed on lower eyelid.
- Left *in situ* for 5 min.

- The distance that any moisture on the paper has spread is recorded.
- >10 mm of wet paper = normal.

Human leucocyte antigen (HLA)

- In ankylosing spondylitis, up to 90% of those affected are positive for HLA-B27. However, up to 2% of the 'normal' population also have positive titres.
- Therefore not everyone with HLA B27 positivity will progress to the disease. Therefore they should only be tested for if there is a high pre-test probability of the disease.

Diseases associated with HLA

A1, B8, DR3	Polymyositis/dermatomyositis
A3; B14	Haemochromatosis
B5	Polycystic kidney disease (PKD), ulcerative colitis (UC), Behçet's syndrome
B8; DR3	Autoimmune hepatitis, Graves' disease, Addison's disease, Sjögren's syndrome, dermatitis herpetiformis, systemic lupus erythematosus (SLE)
B8; DR3; DR7	Coeliac disease
B27	Seronegative spondylarthritides (negative for rheumatoid factor), e.g. ankylosing spondylitis, Reiter's syndrome, psoriatic arthropathy
C6; B13; B17	Psoriasis
DR4; DR3	Type 1 diabetes mellitus
DR5	Hashimoto's thyroiditis Systemic sclerosis

Synovial fluid analysis

- This is the fluid that fills synovial joint cavities in order to reduce friction between joint surfaces.

- Synovial fluid, an ultrafiltrate of plasma, can be needle aspirated.
- Inflammatory and infective conditions often result in an increased volume of fluid, with varying degrees of white cell elevation.

Condition	Leucocyte count (/mm³)	Appearance
Normal	<200	Clear
Gout	3000–40,000	Cloudy, needle-shaped negatively birefringent crystals (sodium urate)
Pseudogout	3000–40,000	Cloudy, rhomboid-shaped weakly positively birefringent crystals (sodium pyrophosphate)
Septic arthritis	>750,000	Murky, purulent

X-ray changes in rheumatological disease

■ Different disease processes affect joints in subtly different ways, producing characteristic appearances on X-ray.

■ Serial X-rays can provide evidence of disease progression.

Disease	Changes on film
Osteoarthritis (Figure 9.1)	Osteophytes; joint space narrowing; bone cysts; subarticular sclerosis
Rheumatoid arthritis (Figure 9.2)	– Soft tissue swelling; decreased joint space; juxta-articular osteoporosis – Late changes: bony erosions, subluxation of joints – Other: cervical spine instability (increased distance between odontoid peg (axis) and anterior arch of atlas on lateral view); pleural effusion/nodules/fibrosing alveolitis on chest X-ray NB: X-ray changes usually manifest quite late in the disease so they should not be used as a criteria for diagnosis and delay of treatment
Gout (Figure 9.3)	Periarticular erosion; soft tissue swelling but no loss of joint space
Osteoporosis (Figure 9.4)	Osteopaenia; healing of previous osteoporotic fractures

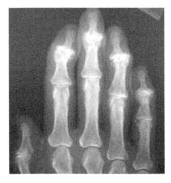

Figure 9.1: Osteoarthritis

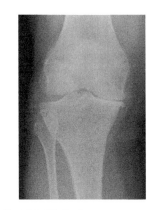

Figure 9.4: Osteoporosis

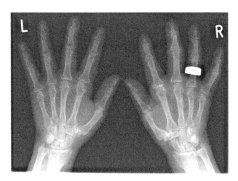

Figure 9.2: Rheumatoid arthritis

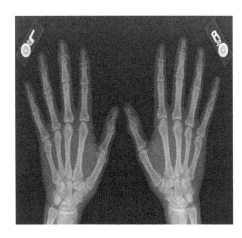

Figure 9.3: Gout

Chapter 10
OBSTETRICS AND GYNAECOLOGY

Introduction

Obstetrics and gynaecology incorporates a unique mix of medical and surgical management of patients. This chapter provides an overview of some of the more common investigation-related topics that appear in examinations. Much of this chapter follows closely from other chapters, for example the sections on hormones (Chapter 5) and imaging techniques used in antenatal screening (Chapter 15).

Topics covered
■ Sex hormones and the menstrual cycle
■ Polycystic ovarian syndrome (PCOS)
■ Infertility
■ Pregnancy testing
■ Antenatal tests
■ Physiological changes of pregnancy
■ Cardiotocography (CTG)

Sex hormones and the menstrual cycle

Luteinising hormone (LH) and follicle-stimulating hormone (FSH)

NB: More details about the hypothalamic-pituitary axis can be found in Chapter 5.

Gonadal hormones

■ Steroid sex hormones are important in inducing primary and secondary sexual characteristics. The key classes are:
• androgens (e.g. testosterone, dihydrotestosterone)
• oestrogens (e.g. oestradiol, oestrione)
• progestagens (e.g. progesterone, progestins).

■ Sex hormone-binding globulin (SHBG) is produced by the liver and binds to the sex hormones testosterone and oestradiol to allow their circulation in the bloodstream. Although only small proportions travel unbound (free), these constitute the 'active' hormone.

■ Levels of SHBG are reduced by insulin, insulin-like growth factor 1 (IGF-1) and high androgen levels, as well as the liver's fat production, e.g. in polycystic ovarian syndrome, diabetes and hypothyroidism.

■ Levels are increased by high oestrogen and thyroxine levels, e.g. in pregnancy, hyperthyroidism and anorexia nervosa.

The hands-on guide to data interpretation. By S. Abraham, K. Kulkarni, R. Madhu and D. Provan. Published 2010 by Blackwell Publishing Ltd.

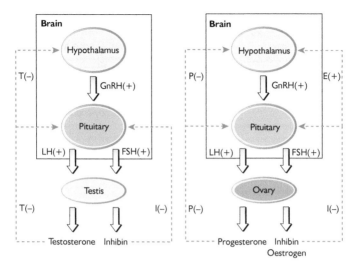

Figure 10.1: Control of sex hormones by the hypothalamic-pituitary axis

Menstrual cycle

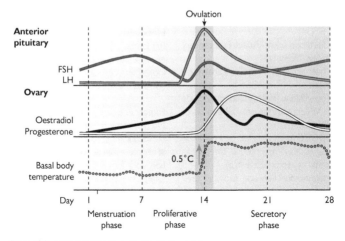

Figure 10.2: Hormonal changes during the menstrual cycle

■ The menstrual cycle usually lasts 28 days and consists of several phases:
• menstrual (days 1–4)
■ follicular (proliferative) (days 5–13)
• ovulation (day 14)
• luteal (secretory) (day 15–26)
• ischaemic (part of secretory) (days 27–28).
■ The follicular phase involves oestrogen-induced endometrial thickening
■ Menstruation occurs for approximately 3–5 days.
■ Most fertile period = days 10–19 pre-menstruation (peak = LH surge).

Menstrual disorders

These can be classified into 'functional' (an organic abnormality) and 'dysfunctional' (assumed due to endocrine disturbance due to lack of any noticeable organic cause). 'AUB' as coined by the NICE Guidelines (2007) refers to 'abnormal uterine bleeding' and includes dysfunctional bleeds.

Investigation of menorrhagia (heavy/abnormal bleeding)
■ Bloods:
• full blood count (?anaemia secondary to heavy bleeding)
• haematinics (iron studies if anaemia is present)
• coagulation (clotting) screen (exclude von Willebrand disease, ITP and factor deficiencies)
• β-hCG (pregnancy can be a common cause of abnormal uterine bleeding in patients of reproductive age)
• thyroid function and prolactin level (excludes thyroid and pituitary causes)
• liver/renal function tests (if dysfunction of either organ suspected, e.g. polycystic ovarian syndrome, alcoholic liver disease)

• hormone assays (LH, FSH, androgen levels if polycystic ovarian syndrome suspected; adrenal function test if adrenal tumour suspected).
■ Ultrasound scan, to visualise any uterine anomaly (e.g. fibroids) or adnexal pathology (e.g. ovarian cyst).
■ A hysteroscopy/endometrial biopsy may be required especially for perimenopausal women. A pipelle device can be used for obtaining an endometrial biopsy in an outpatient setting.
■ Other imaging (e.g. computed tomography (CT) or magnetic resonance imaging (MRI) of pituitary fossa if tumour detected).

Investigation of post-menopausal bleeding
■ An ultrasound scan (USS) is the initial investigation.
■ Endometrial biopsy is required only if the endometrial thickness is over 4 mm on USS.

Investigation of amenorrhoea (lack of normal menstrual bleeding)
Remember that history is important, for example taking into account often overlooked features such as excessive exercise and anorexia nervosa as causes.

Primary amenorrhoea
No menarche by age 16 years, or 14 if no secondary sexual characteristics.
■ Anatomical/constitutional: examination for Turner's syndrome (gonadal failure), imperforate hymen, family history of 'normal' but delayed menarche.
■ Endocrine blood tests:
• thyroid function
• hormone levels – elevated prolactin levels (caused by drugs, tumour, etc.);

testosterone (polycystic ovarian syndrome, androgen insensitivity); LH/FSH (polycystic ovarian syndrome)
• β-hCG (exclude pregnancy)
• congenital adrenal hyperplasia, hypothalamic failure.

■ Pelvic ultrasound scan (confirm presence of uterus, exclude outflow tract obstruction, polycystic ovarian syndrome).

■ Other imaging (e.g. CT/MRI of pituitary fossa if tumour detected).

■ Karyotyping: consider if either uterus or secondary sexual characteristics absent.

Secondary amenorrhoea

Normal menarche commences, but then menstrual cycle stops.
■ Investigations as above. Causes include:
• androgen excess present: polycystic ovarian syndrome (see below), Cushing's syndrome or congenital adrenal hyperplasia (see Chapter 5 for investigation), or adrenal/ovarian malignancy (imaging)
• no androgen excess: history and examination for physiological causes (pregnancy, lactation, menopause), contraceptive use, weight loss (e.g. anorexia) and anatomical (cervical stenosis/intrauterine adhesions – Asherman's syndrome). Serum hormone blood tests for premature ovarian failure (i.e. before age 40) and pituitary disease (hyperprolactinaemia).

Karyotyping

This is a useful investigation in certain cases, and can confirm the presence of several conditions, including the following.

■ Secondary sexual characteristics absent:
• short stature and high FSH and LH suggest gonadal agenesis, e.g. Turner's syndrome
• short stature and low FSH and LH suggest an intracranial lesion, e.g. hydrocephalus, trauma to skull, tumour (craniopharyngioma)
• normal height and high FSH and LH suggest premature ovarian failure if karyotype is normal, and 46XY agenesis or XY enzymatic failure if karyotype is abnormal.
• normal height and low FSH and LH suggest hypogonadotrophic hypogonadism, e.g. Kallmann's syndrome.

■ Uterus absent:
• 46XX: Meyer-Rokitansky-Kuster-Hauser syndrome: normal external female genitalia but rudimentary uterine development
• 46XY: XY female, e.g. androgen insensitivity syndrome.

NB: For more information on endocrinological conditions such as hypothalamic failure, intersex, congenital adrenal hyperplasia, etc., please see Chapter 5.

Polycystic ovarian syndrome (PCOS)

■ In this syndrome, the ovaries are larger and have an abnormal number of small follicles (cystic).

■ The lack of normal development leads to ovulatory failure and subfertility.

■ The menstrual cycle is correspondingly irregular or infrequent (oligomenorrhoea). Other features include acne, hirsutism, obesity and insulin resistance.

Investigation

Diagnosis is based on the following criteria.

■ Clinic features of PCOS (e.g. oligo/anovulation, signs of hyperandrogenism).

■ Ultrasound: usually trans-vaginal, to directly examine for presence of:

• polycystic ovaries (usually >12 peripheral follicles on each ovary, each not exceeding 10 mm in size and being relatively immature)

• increased ovarian volume (>10 cm^3).

■ Blood:

• elevated LH in the early part of the cycle (raised LH/FSH ratio is often seen, although is not strictly part of the diagnostic criteria due to it's inconsistency)

• elevated androgens (testosterone, androstenedione, 5-dehydroepiandrosterone (5-DHEA))

• lower sex-hormone binding globulin

• lower day 21 progesterone

• elevated glucose or impaired oral glucose tolerance test (PCOS is associated with insulin resistance; see Chapter 5 for more details).

NB: Other baseline tests include: HDL cholesterol (often low), prolactin (elevated), and free androgen index (total testosterone/SHBG). A diagnosis can only be made when other aetiologies have been excluded (e.g. hyperthyroidism, androgen-secreting tumours, Cushing's syndrome, congenital adrenal hyperplasia (elevated 17-hydroxyprogesterone), etc.).

Remember the following.

1 A finding of PCO on USS without any of the remaining two criteria is not synonymous with PCOS.

2 Amenorrhoea for >3 months can result in an increased risk of endometrial malignancy due to the hyper-oestrogenic state that characterises this condition. Hence, patients should be advised on inducing a withdrawal bleed if amenorrhoea lasts >3 months.

Withdrawal bleeds

■ There is a link between severe oligo- and amenorrhoea in the presence of pre-menopausal oestrogen levels, and endometrial hyperplasia and carcinoma.

■ In particular, intervals between menstruations of more than 3 months may be associated with endometrial hyperplasia.

■ Therefore amenorrhoeic or severely oligomenorrhoeic women with PCOS should have induced withdrawal bleeds at regular intervals to reduce the risk of developing endometrial hyperplasia.

■ Withdrawal bleeds can be induced with cyclical progestogens (for at least 12 days), with oral contraceptive pills, or by use of the Mirena intrauterine system.

Infertility

For investigative purposes, the causes of infertility can be divided into: male, anovulatory and tubal factors.

Male

■ Physical/psychological factors:

• these should be elicited with a thorough history and clinical examination

• for example paraplegia, Peyronie's disease, depression, etc.

■ Semen factors:

• normal: volume >2 mL, sperm count >20,000/mL, sperm motility >50%, abnormal forms <20%; pH > 7.2

• these normal values can vary between individuals (i.e. men can still be fertile despite not fulfilling the above criteria), and at least three specimens should be examined in any case.
■ Hormonal factors:
• low LH/FSH
• low testosterone (consider chromosome analysis if count <5,000,000/mL).

Anovulatory (female)

This can occur in up to 10% of regularly menstruating women. Investigations include the following.
■ Temperature chart: usually a fall pre-ovulation followed by a sustained 0.3–0.5°C rise during luteal phase. This, however, is often a source of anxiety for patients, and basal body temperature monitoring is not recommended by NICE on the grounds that it is not a reliable marker of ovulation.
■ Hormone assays: elevated day 21 serum progesterone usually means ovulation has occurred, although false-positives can occur with luteinisation of a follicle, so this is usually combined with ultrasound. The test should ideally be done 7 days prior to the onset of menstruation (hence with a 32-day cycle it should be done on day 25). Also check for elevated prolactin on more than one occasion (again, false-positives can occur), as well as LH/FSH (altered ratio or chronic elevation in polycystic ovarian disease), and thyroid function.
■ Ultrasound: observe growth of follicles during day 8–18 of cycle (one should grow >20mm). Note that this is undertaken in specialist assisted conception units.
■ Endometrial biopsy: can be performed 1–3 days pre-menstrually to check for secretory changes. Not commonly performed.

Tubal (female)

This can be investigated using the following techniques.
■ Laparoscopy and dye insufflation: one of the more commonly used investigations to visualise the tubes and ovaries. Hysteroscopy is also commonly performed at the same time to exclude polyps and submucous fibroids, as well as intra-uterine adhesions.
■ Hysterosalpingogram: insertion of contrast through the cervix and imaging with X-rays to visualise the shape of the uterus and patency of the fallopian tubes.

Pregnancy testing

■ Modern pregnancy tests are based on the detection of β-hCG (human chorionic gonadotrophin) in urine samples. These detect levels between 20 and 100mIU/mL.
■ False-negatives occur, particularly with early testing.
■ Serum samples can also be used for analysis by enzyme-linked immunosorbant assay (ELISA) for the presence of β-HCG. These are more sensitive than urine assays and can detect levels as low as 1mIU/mL.
■ Positivity for β-hCG usually occurs 6–12 days after fertilisation.
■ Ultrasound detection of a gestational sac is usually positive from 4½ weeks post-gestation (2½ weeks after ovulation). A heartbeat is usually detected at between 6 and 7 weeks of gestation.

Antenatal tests

There are number of investigations that can be undertaken during pregnancy to screen for a range of abnormalities. In the UK, these include the following.

■ Basic blood investigations:
• blood group
• rhesus factor (anti-D should be administered to those found to be Rh negative)
• full blood count
• infections: syphilis, hepatitis B, rubella, HIV
• random glucose/glucose tolerance test (usually only if suspected gestational diabetes – not routinely performed)
• electrophoresis for sickle-cell and thalassaemia (haemoglobinopathy screening is relevant in at-risk populations, e.g. Mediterranean, African descent).
■ Amniocentesis (amniotic fluid sampling) (15th–18th week):
• chromosomal disorders (e.g. Down syndrome) – amniocentesis is only offered to screen positive patients
• neural tube defects (e.g. spina bifida) – this is an ultrasound scan diagnosis, although elevated alpha-fetoprotein (AFP) can also occur
• determining sex of foetus – again, usually detected on scan (amniocentesis is therefore not used primarily for this).
■ Chorionic villus sampling (10th–12th week):
• chromosomal abnormalities (e.g. Down syndrome).
■ Urine (first antenatal visit):
• asymptomatic bacteriuria (risk of pyelonephritis).
■ Ultrasound: in most centres two scans are done: a dating (12 week) and an anomaly (20 week) scan:
• used throughout pregnancy to visualise development of foetus:
– 6 weeks: intra-uterine sac visible
– 8–10 weeks: gestation sac, foetus (measure 'crown–rump' length) and foetal heart movements

– 12 weeks: gross foetal abnormalities (e.g. anencephaly)
– 16 weeks: sufficient fluid for amniocentesis
– 16–20 weeks: gestational age assessment, assessment of gross anatomical abnormality (e.g. spine, head, abdomen)
– 30–40 weeks: foetal size (e.g. foetal-trunk area, placental site)
■ Foetal anomaly scan (20 weeks):
• this can detect a range of abnormalities, including anencephaly (99%), exomphalos/gastroschisis (90%), major limb abnormalities (90%) and spina bifida (90%)
• ultrasound markers of chromosomal abnormalities are not very sensitive or specific for pathology, but can suggest the need for repeat scanning later in pregnancy, or further investigation such as amniocentesis. Single markers are often insignificant. Markers include:
– renal pelvic dilatation (mild hydronephrosis): a poor marker for Down syndrome (often present in a normal foetus)
– echogenic foci in bowel or cardiac ventricles: in the bowel, this may suggest conditions such as cystic fibrosis
– choroid plexus cysts (CPC): 1% of foetuses have one or more CPCs in early pregnancy, so in the absence of other markers, isolated CPCs are insignificant. They can be a marker for conditions such as Edward's syndrome
– other, more specific markers are often described, for conditions such as Down syndrome (e.g. short femur/humerus, nuchal fold thickness) – see below for more information.

Down syndrome

■ General incidence is 1:1000.
■ The risk by maternal age:
• age 35 = 1:365

- age 40 = 1:109
- age 45 = 1:32.

■ Risk of recurrence is 1% (0.75% higher than maternal age-related risk.

■ In case of parental aneuploidy there is a 30% risk of trisomy in offspring.

■ Summary of tests for Down syndrome:

during first trimester (11–14 weeks)

- nuchal translucency (ultrasound, measure of skin fold thickness behind cervical spine, caused by venous or lymphatic engorgement – 82% detection rate for trisomy 21)
- blood tests: free β-hCG) or pregnancy associated plasma protein A (PAPP-A, Down syndrome)
- chorionic villus sampling or amniocentesis (offered if risk >1 in 250, i.e. high risk pregnancy)

during second trimester (15–20 weeks)

- double test (elevated β-hCG and alpha-fetoprotein (AFP))
- triple test (above, plus oestriol (uE3))
- quadruple test (above, plus inhibin A)

combined first and second trimester screening

- serum integrated test – first trimester: PAPP-A; second trimester: β-hCG, AFP, uE3, inhibin A
- integrated – first trimester: nuchal translucency and PAPP-A, second trimester: β-hCG, uE3, inhibin A, AFP.

Foetal blood sampling

■ Percutaneous umbilical cord blood sampling (PUBS) can be used to obtain sample of foetal blood during pregnancy.

■ The procedure is similar to amniocentesis, and can be used to undertake a chromosome analysis.

■ It is usually performed after 17 weeks.

Foetal scalp blood testing

■ This is a transvaginal procedure performed during labour.

■ It can be used to obtain a sample of blood for pH testing to detect foetal acidaemia, and may indicate foetal hypoxia:

- pH 7.25 = normal (allow labour to continue)
- pH 7.–7.25 = borderline (if delivery is anticipated within 1–2 h, repeat within 1 h)
- pH <7.2 = abnormal, deliver immediately.

NB: PUBS and scalp blood sampling are usually contraindicated in cases of maternal infection (e.g. HIV, hepatitis, herpes simplex), foetal bleeding disorders (e.g. haemophilia, low platelets) and prematurity (<34 weeks gestation).

Antenatal ultrasound

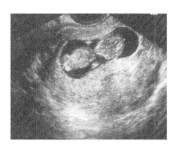

Figure 10.3: Normal intrauterine pregnancy

Foetal cardiology scans

■ Congenital heart disease is one of the commonest malformations, affecting approximately 1% neonates.

■ Foetal echocardiography can be undertaken alongside other anomaly scanning, usually between 18 and 23 weeks gestation.

■ This is particularly of benefit in those at high risk, e.g. those with a family history of congenital heart disease, maternal drug use (e.g. anti-epileptic drugs, lithium), increased nuchal translucency/presence of other foetal malformations (e.g. exomphalos) and maternal diabetes mellitus.

Physiological changes of pregnancy

A number of normal changes can occur in the mother during pregnancy. They include the following.

Cardiovascular

■ Full blood count: haemoglobin can be lower due to a dilutional effect caused by a greater blood volume (especially plasma volume).

■ Other blood constituents: raised red cell mass, increased fibrinogen and platelet counts, increased factors VII, X, XII.

■ Blood volume: this increases from 6–8 weeks gestation and reaches a maximum around 32–34 weeks.

■ Blood pressure: slight fall in diastolic pressure by mid-pregnancy. Due to an increased sympathetic control of BP and increased venous distension, hypotension can develop more readily (a more 'hyper-dynamic' circulation).

■ Aorto-caval compression: the uterus compresses the descending aorta and the inferior vena cava, thus impeding venous return.

■ Cardiac output: this initially increases proportionally to match the increased blood volume. However, with greater aorto-caval compression towards term,

cardiac output can fall. Increased stroke volume, systemic vascular resistance and heart rate usually compensate this for.

■ All of these factors are particularly of relevance during trauma – be this acute injury or during procedures such as surgery. For example, lower volumes of local anaesthetic are required to achieve similar blocks (compared with non-pregnant women). To maintain venous return, shifting the foetus (by lying on the left side when supine, for example) can help reduce the effects of aorto-caval compression.

Respiratory

■ Lung volumes: although the foetus causes diaphragmatic elevation, this is compensated for by corresponding increases in antero-posterior and transverse chest diameters. Expiratory reserve volume, functional residual volume and residual volume decrease midway through the second trimester. Tidal volume increases by up to 40%.

■ Minute ventilation: this increases at an early stage and reaches a level 50% above normal during the second trimester, and is accompanied by a rise in respiratory rate of 2–3 breaths/min. Oxygen consumption increases to accommodate the needs of the foetus (up to 20% normal).

■ Arterial blood gases: average PaO_2 = 13.7 kPa (105 mmHg) and average $PaCO_2$ = 4.3 kPa (32 mmHg).

■ Another important point to note is an increased risk of aspiration (largely due to a combination of the compression of the abdominal contents caused by the foetus, and a relaxation of the stomach sphincters and slower gastric emptying times).

■ All of these factors can be summarised as increased oxygen consumption and decreased reserve capacity, i.e. reduced compensatory ability in the event of hypoxia.

Renal

■ Glomerular filtration rate (GFR): this increases considerably, alongside renal plasma flow (both up to 50%).

■ Urea and creatinine: the levels of these decrease correspondingly (up to 40%).

■ Plasma osmolality: water retention leads to a decrease in this.

■ Protein and glucose: both of these can be present in mild amounts (up to 10 g/day glucose and 300 mg/day protein).

Endocrine

■ Metabolic rate: broadly speaking, global metabolic demands increase during pregnancy, i.e. increased basal metabolic rate.

■ Glucose: symptoms of hypoglycaemia may commence at a lower level than in non-pregnant women, due to restricted autonomic compensatory mechanisms. Maternal serum glucose levels are also generally lower after an overnight fast as compared with non-pregnant women.

Cardiotocography (CTG)

■ This is a method of externally (non-invasively) recording the foetal heartbeat and uterine contractions.

■ It is used during labour to identify foetal distress (which may require prompt delivery).

■ Correspondingly, there are usually two tracings: the upper tracing is usually the foetal heartbeat, while the lower tracing records uterine contractions.

■ Different aspects of the tracing can yield information about the status of the foetus. For example:

• baseline rate (usually between 110–160 bpm)

• baseline variability of 5–15 bpm

• accelerations (sustained increase >15 bpm for at least 15 s) are suggesting of normal foetal activity and are not usually pathological

• decelerations (sustained decreases >15 bpm for at least 15 s) can be normal. However, when they occur later (after contractions), they can suggest foetal distress. Variability in deceleration patterns can suggest other pathologies such as hypoxia

• bradycardia (slowing <100 bpm) for over 3 min is an abnormal feature

• tachycardia (speeds >160 bpm) can be suggestive of foetal infection or pyrexia, as well as other causes of foetal distress. Hypovolaemia and maternal tachycardia can also cause foetal tachycardia.

■ Abnormal CTGs require ongoing monitoring of mother and foetus, as well as further investigation. This can include more invasive procedures such as foetal blood sampling.

NB: bpm = beats per minute.

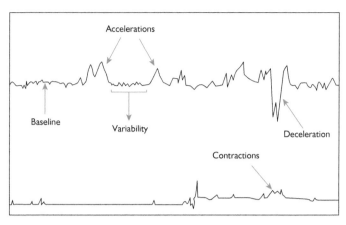

Figure 10.4: Changes seen on cardiotocography

Chapter 11
OPHTHALMOLOGY

Introduction

The eye is not only home to a vast array of pathologies of its own, but can also be a window to systemic pathology. This chapter covers only the fundamentals of eye-related investigations. While further assessment of visual function is often confined to neurological examination of the relevant cranial nerves, it is important to be aware of the other investigative modalities available. With fundoscopy being the commonest bedside ophthalmological investigation that students and junior doctors are likely to encounter, we have included a number of labelled fundoscopy images of key pathologies. Beyond this, we will briefly consider several other eye-imaging modalities and discuss techniques for more detailed assessment of visual fields and acuity. Further consideration of various ophthalmological pathologies can be found in the relevant sections of other chapters.

Topics covered
- Fundoscopy
- Other eye imaging modalities
- Assessment of visual acuity
- Assessment of visual fields
- Corneal topography

Fundoscopy

- Fundoscopy (ophthalmoscopy) can be used to visualise various layers of the eye.
- This allows examination of the posterior pole, including the retinal blood vessels, the optic disc and parts of the retina, including the macula.
- The ophthalmoscope also allows the 'red reflex' to be seen (glow from choroid). This can be reduced or absent with a number of pathologies, including cataract, tumours and intraocular haemorrhage.
- Refractive error (your own and that of the patient) can be corrected using the dials on the ophthalmoscope: + corrects hypermetropia or 'long' sight (able to see distant objects clearly); − corrects myopia or 'short' sight (able to see close objects clearly).
- The examination should ideally take place in a darkened room, with glasses removed and, if required, with a mydriatic (e.g. tropicamide) to dilate the pupil.
- A slit lamp is a fixed device that allows detailed examination of all parts of the eye. It also facilitates intraocular pressure measurement (tonometry); see below for more details.
- The following images demonstrate some of the more common ophthalmological pathologies.

The hands-on guide to data interpretation. By S. Abraham, K. Kulkarni, R. Madhu and D. Provan. Published 2010 by Blackwell Publishing Ltd.

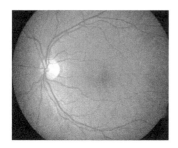

Figure 11.1: Normal left eye

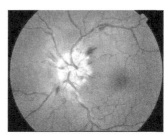

Figure 11.4: Papilloedema

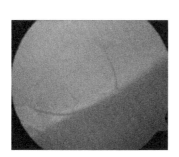

Figure 11.2: Retinal detachment

Flame haemorrhages

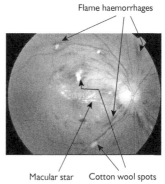

Macular star   Cotton wool spots

Figure 11.5: Hypertensive retinopathy (grade 3)

Temporal disc pallor

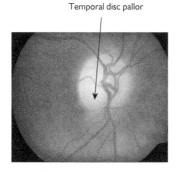

Figure 11.3: Optic atrophy

Microaneurysms

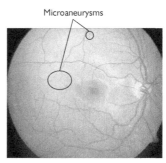

Figure 11.6: Background diabetic retinopathy

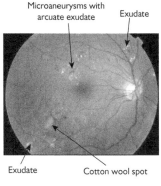

Microaneurysms with arcuate exudate

Exudate

Exudate

Cotton wool spot

Figure 11.7: Diabetic retinopathy

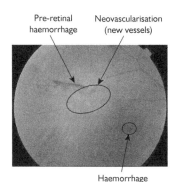

Pre-retinal haemorrhage

Neovascularisation (new vessels)

Haemorrhage

Figure 11.8: New vessel proliferation (angiogenesis)

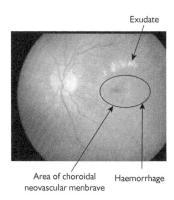

Exudate

Area of choroidal neovascular menbrave

Haemorrhage

Figure 11.9: Exudative age-related macular generation

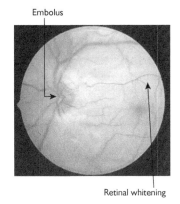

Embolus

Retinal whitening

Figure 11.10: Central retinal artery occlusion

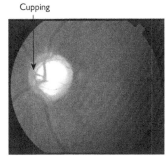

Cupping

Figure 11.11: Disc cupping in glaucoma

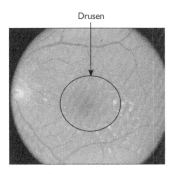

Drusen

Figure 11.12: Drusen

Other eye imaging modalities

Slit lamp examination

■ This allows binocular examination of the eye using a high-intensity light source system and a microscope.

■ It allows examination of the anterior and posterior segment of the eye, including the eyelid, sclera, conjunctiva, iris, lens and cornea.

■ Mydriatics and fluorescein may be applied to the eye to aid examination. Fluorescein can help visualise corneal defects.

■ Pathologies that can be visualised, are similar to those that can be seen with fundoscopy.

■ The procedure requires the patient to rest their chin on the headrest, and to align their eyes to look straight into the microscope.

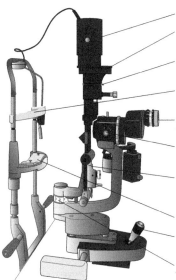

Lamp (light bulb)

Calibrated scale for measuring length of light beam (and lesions)

Disc for adjusting brightness of beam and for applying filters (e.g. cobalt blue)

Patient forehead strap (rest forehead here)

Eyepieces (oculars)–examiner looks through here–(similar to binoculars)

Lever/knob for adjusting magnification (strength usually up to 25x)

Illumination arm–can be rotated 180° sideways to examine from the nasal to the temporal aspects of the eye

Patient rests chin here

Joystick for adjusting the position of the viewing and illuminating arms

Knobs for adjusting the width of light beam

Figure 11.13: Components of a slit lamp

Retinal photography

■ This technique allows the state of the retina to be recorded and compared over time.

■ It is of use in any chronic condition causing retinal changes, such as diabetic

retinopathy or age-related macular degeneration.

Fluorescein angiography

■ This involves sequential photography of the retina after intravenous sodium fluorescein administration.

■ This is of use in visualising microvascular changes in detail, including ischaemia, neovascularisation and leakage from blood vessels.

■ It can determine what treatment may be appropriate.

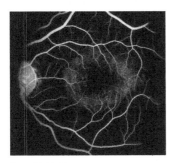

Figure 11.14: Fluorescein angiogram

Indocyanine green angiography

■ This is similar to fluorescein angiography but uses a different intravenous dye.

■ It allows imaging of choroidal pathology.

Optical coherence tomography

■ Light interferometry is used to produce a cross-sectional representation of the layers of the retina.

■ This is extremely useful in diagnosis and monitoring of macular pathology, including macular oedema, macular holes and age-related macular degeneration.

Visual acuity

Visual acuity is a measure of central vision. It is commonly assessed by the use of a Snellen chart.

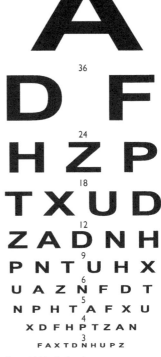

Figure 11.15: Snellen chart

■ Patient should sit 6 m from the chart. Distances can be compensated for in small rooms by the use of mirrors or reduced charts.

■ The chart is designed with a series of a letters in descending order of size.

■ The top line is a size that can be read by someone with normal vision at 60 m. The second line can be read by someone with normal vision at 36 m. This continues down the chart, giving a series of acuity measures.

■ The top number is the distance from the chart, the second is the distance at which the particular line 'should' be read by an individual with normal vision:

- 6/60 (top line)
- 6/36
- 6/24
- 6/18
- 6/12
- 6/9
- 6/6 (bottom line).

■ Normal vision is considered to be 6/6.

■ If an individual has difficulty reading the top line (i.e. worse than 6/60 vision), then the distance from the chart can be progressively reduced (e.g. initially from 6 m → 5 m). The measurement is adjusted accordingly (e.g. if the top line can only be read at 4 m, then the acuity would be '4/60').

■ For vision worse than 6/6, a pin-hole can be used (essentially a tiny hole in a piece of paper). As this removes the need for focusing, straightforward refractive errors should be corrected. If other ocular pathologies are the cause of the visual loss, this may not correct the loss of acuity.

■ If vision is below 1/60, the patient can be asked to count the examiner's fingers ('CF' measurement) at a distance of ½ m.

■ Below this, 'HM' (hand movements seen), 'PL' (perception of light) or 'NPL' (no perception of light) can be recorded.

LogMAR chart (Figure 11.16)

■ The more accurate Keeler logMAR test has become increasingly popular, replacing the Snellen chart in both clinical and research environments.

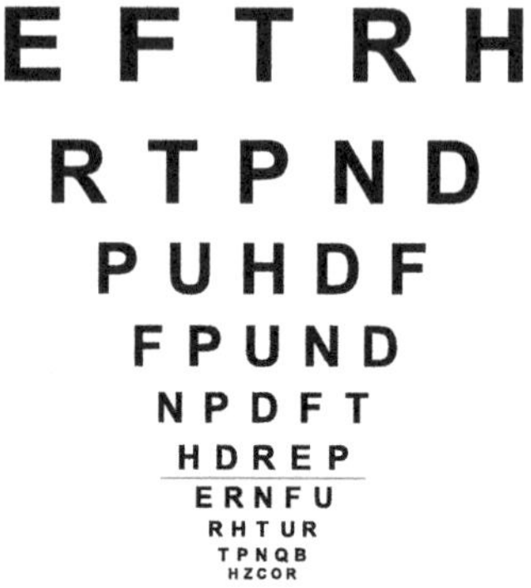

E F T R H
R T P N D
P U H D F
F P U N D
N P D F T
H D R E P
E R N F U
R H T U R
T P N Q B
H Z C O R

Figure 11.16: LogMAR chart

■ This uses letters of particular font (with lines of equal thickness), with letters spaced at regular intervals. Letter size progression is uniform.

■ Advantages include an equal number of letters per line, and a greater overall number of letters per line than the Snellen chart, allowing a greater range of assessment for those with poorer acuity.

■ It involves the logarithm (to base 10) of the width (minutes of arc) of the limbs of a letter. Each letter is scored individually (each letter scores 0.025), allowing for a more accurate 'total scoring of visual acuity.

Visual fields

Perimetry

■ This is the measure of differential light sensitivity in the peripheral or central visual field.

■ It can be useful in the investigation of a number of ocular and neurological conditions.

■ The pattern of visual field defect can be used to localise the likely pathology.

■ The patient is required to detect various targets on a defined background.

■ Static perimetry (e.g. Humphrey) places targets of differing intensities at different points on the visual field. Kinetic perimetry (e.g. Goldmann) brings stimuli from the periphery to the centre until they are detected.

■ The central visual field can be mapped using an Amsler grid. The patient is instructed to look at the central dot with the fellow eye closed. They are then asked to draw the border of the area that they cannot see.

■ Distortion of the lines of an Amsler grid can be seen in certain macular pathology, such as age-related macular degeneration.

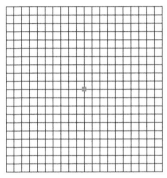 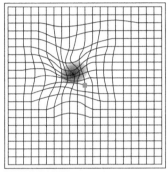

Normal vision   Age-related macular degeneration

Figure 11.17: Amsler grids

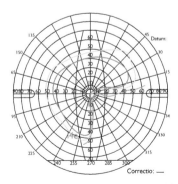

Figure 11.18: Goldmann field – demonstrates a missing upper temporal field

Corneal topography

■ Also known as photokeratoscopy. This is a non-invasive technique for mapping the surface curvature of the cornea.

■ It is of use in the investigation of refractive errors.

■ A topographer consists of a lit bowl (which the patient looks into). This displays a series of concentric rings that are focused on the anterior surface of the patient's cornea and are reflected back to a camera.

■ The reflected pattern can then be used to produce a topographical map, colour coding the curvature by dioptric value (optical power). Maps can be in different planes, including axial (power or sagittal map – the standard output), tangential (uses different mathematical calculations and does not assume that the eye is spherical), elevation and refractive.

■ Indications for topography include the investigation of suspected keratoconus. It is also of benefit pre/post-surgery, particularly in patients who have undergone penetrating keratoplasty, radial keratotomy or LASIK. In these patients, corneal maps can assist with pre-operative planning, as well as postoperative healing assessment and contact lens fitting.

Chapter 12
ONCOLOGY

Introduction

Cancer, the unregulated growth of tissues, continues to bear an increasing influence on all specialties. While the other chapters in this book consider cancers relevant to a particular system, this section will discuss the basics of oncology. With a raft of essential terminology to be aware of, this chapter provides a framework to approaching the investigation and management of specific cancers.

Topics covered
- Cancer statistics
- Language of cancer therapy
- Screening
- Tumour markers
- Tumour stage and grade

Cancer statistics

- In the UK each year a quarter of a million people will be diagnosed with cancer and over 150,000 people will die as a result.
- The following table shows figures for the 'top 10' cancers.

	Cancer mortality (2005)			Cancer incidence (2004)		
Rank	All (n)	Males	Females	All (n)	Males	Females
1	Lung (33,465)	Lung	Lung	Breast (44,659)	Prostate	Breast
2	Colorectal (16,092)	Prostate	Breast	Lung (38,313)	Lung	Colorectal
3	Breast (12,509)	Colorectal	Colorectal	Colorectal (36,109)	Colorectal	Lung
4	Prostate (10,000)	Oesophagus	Ovary	Prostate (34,986)	Bladder	Ovary
5	Gastric (7,419)	Gastric	Pancreas	Bladder (10,093)	Non-Hodgkin's lymphoma	Uterine

(Continued)

The hands-on guide to data interpretation. By S. Abraham, K. Kulkarni, R. Madhu and D. Provan. Published 2010 by Blackwell Publishing Ltd.

(Continued)

Rank	Cancer mortality (2005)			Cancer incidence (2004)		
	All (n)	Males	Females	All (n)	Males	Females
6	Pancreas (7,238)	Pancreas	Oesophagus	Non-Hodgkin's lymphoma (10,003)	Gastric	Melanoma
7	Stomach (5,672)	Bladder	Gastric	Melanoma (8,939)	Oesophagus	Non-Hodgkin's lymphoma
8	Bladder (4,734)	Leukaemia	Non-Hodgkin's lymphoma	Gastric (8,178)	Renal	Pancreas
9	Non-Hodgkin's lymphoma (4,451)	Non-Hodgkin's lymphoma	Leukaemia	Oesophagus (7,654)	Leukaemia	Gastric
10	Ovarian (4,447)	Renal	Uterine	Pancreas (7,398)	Melanoma	Leukaemia

Source: UK Cancer Statistics, Cancer Research UK

Language of cancer therapy

■ *Adjuvant therapy:* treatment given for cancer in the absence of macroscopic evidence of disease after completion of initial therapy (frequently surgery) to patients considered at high risk of recurrence.

■ *Neoadjuvant therapy:* treatment given to tumour that remains in situ prior to initial therapy. Given with the aim of reducing initial tumour size, typically rendering it more amenable to surgery and to treat micrometastasis.

■ *Palliative therapy:* treatment given when cure is not possible, with the intent to prolong survival and relieve symptoms.

Chemotherapy

■ Chemotherapeutic agents are drugs that induce cell death by promotion of apoptosis, commonly by inducing DNA damage or the mitotic spindle apparatus.

■ The following table contains details about some of the more commonly used agents.

Agent	Class	Notable toxicities	Common usages
Cyclophosphamide	Alkylating agent	Myelosuppression, nausea and vomiting, gonadal dysfunction, haemorrhagic cystitis	Breast, non-Hodgkin's lymphoma (NHL), leukaemia
Doxorubicin	Anthracycline antibiotic	Myelosuppression, nausea and vomiting, mucositis, alopecia, acute and chronic cardiac toxicity associated with higher cumulative doses or with other predisposing cardiac factors	Breast, NHL, Hodgkin's, gastric, leukaemia, lung
5-Fluorouracil	Thymidylate synthase inhibitor	Myelosuppression, nausea and vomiting, diarrhoea, and hand foot syndrome	Colorectal, upper gastrointestinal, breast, head and neck
Paclitaxel and docetaxel	Taxanes	Myelosuppression, myalgias and arthralgias, neuropathy, infusion-related reactions	Breast, ovarian, prostate (docetaxel)
Methotrexate	Antifolate	Mucositis, renal impairment, myelosuppression	NHL, leukaemia, choriocarcinoma
Vincristine	Vinca alkaloid	Neurotoxicity, constipation, myelosuppression	NHL, leukaemia
Cisplatin	Platinum compound	Nausea and vomiting, neuropathy, renal dysfunction	Germ cell, ovarian, lung, bladder, upper gastrointestinal
Etoposide	Epipodophyllotoxin	Myelosuppression, mucositis, therapy related myelodysplasia	Leukaemia, small cell lung cancer, ovarian, germ cell
Bleomycin	Antitumour antibiotic	Skin and nail changes, pulmonary toxicity	Germ cell, Hodgkin's

Radiation therapy

■ This is commonly referred to as 'radiotherapy'.
■ It involves the delivery of ionising radiation to affected tissue, which induces DNA strand breakage and apoptosis.
■ Radiation is typically delivered as an external beam generated by a linear accelerator, but may be given by direct contact of the tumour to the radiation source (brachytherapy).

Endocrine therapy

■ This involves modification of the hormonal environment to induce regressions in tumours (e.g. breast and prostrate cancer) whose growth is hormone responsive.

Immunotherapy

■ These are treatments that boost or restore the ability of the immune system to treat cancer.

■ These include monoclonal antibodies (e.g. rituximab in B-cell lymphoma), cytokines (interferon (IFN)-α in renal cell carcinoma) and vaccines.

Small molecules

■ These are a class of drugs that act directly to inhibit the oncogenic proteins driving cancer (e.g. imatinib in chronic myeloid leukaemia (CML) and erlotinib in non-small cell lung cancer).

Screening

■ Screening involves the detection of premalignant/preinvasive conditions (e.g. dysplasia/carcinoma *in situ*), or early malignancy at early asymptomatic stage.

■ By facilitating earlier detection, the aim of screening is to allow early treatment thus preventing cancer-related morbidity and mortality.

Ten principles govern the development of screening programmes as defined by the World Health Organization (WHO).

1 The condition is an important health problem.

2 Its natural history is well understood.

3 It is recognisable at an early stage.

4 Treatment is better at an early stage.

5 A suitable test exists.

6 An acceptable test exists.

7 Adequate facilities exist to cope with abnormalities detected.

8 Screening is done at repeated intervals when the onset is insidious.

9 The chance of harm is less than the chance of benefit.

10 The cost is balanced against benefit. In the UK, screening programmes exist for breast, cervical and bowel malignancies.

Example: breast cancer

■ In the UK, routine screening is offered to all women aged 50–70 years, and occurs every 3 years.

■ With current mammography, 3.7% of screened patients will be required to attend for assessment visit.

■ At the assessment visit 'triple assessment' is used. This comprises:
• clinical examination
• imaging (ultrasound mammography)
• histology (fine needle aspiration/core biopsy), if indicated.

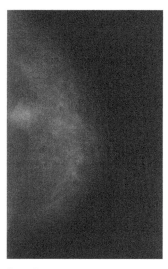

Figure 12.1: Mammogram

Example: cervical cancer

■ In the UK, routine screening is offered to all women aged 25–64 years, and occurs every 3 years (age 25–49) or every 5 years (50–64). The risk of cervical cancer is low in those women who have never been sexually active.

■ It involves a cervical smear. A newer technique utilises liquid-based cytology, a method of preparing samples.

Example: colorectal cancer

■ Roll out nationwide in the UK took place in 2009. A faecal occult blood (FOB) test is posted directly to the patient and returned to area facility by post.

■ It will offer screening to those aged 60–69, every 2 years.

■ If the FOB test is positive, then further assessment and colonoscopy are offered.

Example: prostate cancer

■ There are currently no plans in the UK for a national screening programme for prostate cancer in asymptomatic men, given the criteria for a screening programme in this disease are not yet met.

■ However, there is demand for PSA screening and the current strategy is to give clear balanced advice on the advantages and disadvantages of PSA testing.

Tumour markers

■ Tumour markers are proteins.

■ Cancer is the unregulated growth of normal tissue, hence both malignant and non-malignant tissues produce these proteins.

■ This dramatically reduces their specificity and sensitivity as isolated diagnostic or screening tools.

■ However, when appropriately used alongside clinical findings and other investigations, they can be useful adjuncts in diagnosis, prognostic evaluation, and monitoring treatment response and as markers of recurrence.

Marker	Main malignancy association	Other malignancy associations	Benign pathology associations
AFP	Hepatocellular carcinoma (HCC), non-seminomatous germ-cell tumour (NSGCT)	Gastric, biliary, pancreatic	Cirrhosis, viral hepatitis, pregnancy (especially with spinal cord defects), ataxia-telangiectasia
β-hCG	NSGCT, gestational trophoblastic	Bladder, gastrointestinal (rare)	Pregnancy, gestational trophoblastic disease (GTD), hypogonadism

(Continued)

ONCOLOGY

(Continued)

Marker	Main malignancy association	Other malignancy associations	Benign pathology associations
CA 15-3	Breast	Ovary, lung, HCC	Chronic hepatitis, hepatic cirrhosis, sarcoidosis, tuberculosis (TB), systemic lupus erythematosus (SLE)
CA 19-9	Pancreatic, biliary tree	Colorectal, oesophageal, HCC, gastric	Pancreatitis, biliary disease, cirrhosis
CA-125	Ovarian	Endometrial, fallopian tube, breast, lung, oesophageal, gastric, HCC, pancreatic	Pregnancy, endometriosis, fibroids, ovarian cysts, pelvic inflammation, cirrhosis, pancreatitis, ascites, pleural/pericardial effusion, congestive cardiac failure
CEA	Colorectal	Breast, lung, gastric, pancreatic, thyroid (medullary), head and neck, cervical, hepatic, lymphoma, melanoma	Peptic ulcer disease, inflammatory bowel disease, pancreatitis, hypothyroidism, cirrhosis, biliary obstruction
PSA	Prostate		Prostatitis, benign prostatic hyperplasia (BPH), prostatic trauma, post-ejaculation
5-HIAA	Carcinoid		Certain drugs (e.g. reserpine) and foods (e.g. plums, bananas, etc.), untreated malabsorption
S-100	Melanoma	Peripheral nerve sheath tumours, clear cell sarcomas	Head injury, neurodegenerative disease, cerebrovascular ischaemia

(Continued)

(*Continued*)

Marker	Main malignancy association	Other malignancy associations	Benign pathology associations
Calcitonin	Medullary carcinoma of thyroid	Ectopic tumours (e.g. bronchogenic (lung) carcinoma), breast carcinoma	Post-pentagastrin/ calcium infusion
Thyroglobulin	Papillary and follicular thyroid		Hyperthyroidism (e.g. Graves' disease)
Paraprotein	Myeloma/other B-cell disorders		

Adapted from Kulkarni K, Abraham S, McNeish I (2008) Understanding tumour markers. *Student BMJ* **1**: 35–7.

Tumour stage and grade

■ Staging and grading of tumours is important in determining prognosis and management.

■ Staging = spread (local → distant, degree of lymph node involvement).

■ Grade = degree of differentiation or 'progress' of a tumour ('poorly differentiated' generally means a more aggressive tumour).

Stage

■ Staging of solid tumours is often undertaken using the TNM (tumour, nodes, metastasis) system.

■ This is based on information including clinical examination, imaging (e.g. X-ray, computed tomography (CT)) and procedural findings (e.g. at endoscopy or laparoscopy).

■ Further detail can be added by histological examination of a tumour sample.

■ Certain cancers have their own specific staging systems. For example, lymphoma is staged using the Ann Arbor classification and bowel cancers are staged using Dukes' system.

TNM

■ A number is used for each section to denote the stage of the cancer, e.g. T2N2M0.

■ A higher number denotes a more advanced tumour.

■ The components are:

• tumour (T) = primary tumour (0–4); 'is' can be used to denote '*in situ*'

• nodes (N) = regional lymph node involvement (0–4); 0 = no nodal involvement, 1 = few/local nodes, 3 = many/distant nodes

• metastasis (M) = 0 (no metastasis) or 1 (distant organ metastases present).

NB: An 'X' for any section indicates that evaluation could not take place.

■ Other features:

• c = based on clinical examination

- p = based on pathologic examination
- R (0, 1 or 2): 0 = clear resection-boundaries (free of tumour).

Example: breast carcinoma (TNM)

■ **T:**
- TX: cannot be assessed
- T0: no evidence of primary tumour
- Tis: carcinoma *in situ*, or Paget's disease of the nipple (without detectable tumour mass)
- T1: tumour ≤2 cm (in greatest dimension)
- T2: tumour 2–5 cm (in greatest dimension)
- T3: tumour ≥5 cm (in greatest dimension)
- T4: tumour of any size, with direct spread to chest wall or skin (includes inflammatory carcinoma and ulceration of the breast skin).

■ **N:**
- N0: regional lymph nodes tumour-free
- N1: metastasis to movable, same-side, axillary lymph node(s)
- N2: metastasis to same-side lymph node(s) fixed to one another, or to other structures
- N3: metastasis to same-side lymph nodes beneath the breastbone (internal mammary nodes).

■ **M:**
- MX: the presence of distant metastasis cannot be assessed
- M0: no distant metastases are found
- M1: distant metastases are present.

■ This is sometimes grouped as follows:

- Stage 0: *in situ* breast cancer – Tis, N0, M0
- Stage I: T1, N0, M0
- Stage IIa: T0–1, N1, M0, or T2, N0, M0
- Stage IIb: T2, N1, M0, or T3, N0, M0
- Stage IIIa: T0-2, N2, M0, or T3, N1–2, M0
- Stage IIIb: T4, N (any), M0, or T (any), N3, M0
- Stage IV: T (any), N (any), M1.

Example: colorectal carcinoma (Dukes' system)

■ Primary tumour (T):
- TX: primary tumour cannot be assessed
- T0: no evidence of primary tumour
- Tis: carcinoma *in situ*: intraepithelial or invasion of the lamina propria
- T1: tumour invades submucosa
- T2: tumour invades muscularis propria
- T3: tumour invades through the muscularis propria into the subserosa
- T4: tumour directly invades other organs or structures, and/or perforates visceral peritoneum.

■ Regional lymph nodes (N):
- NX: regional nodes cannot be assessed
- N0: no regional lymph node metastasis
- N1: metastasis in 1 to 3 regional lymph nodes
- N2: metastasis in 4 or more regional lymph nodes

■ Distant metastasis (M):
- MX: distant metastasis cannot be assessed
- M0: no distant metastasis
- M1: distant metastasis.

Stage	T	N	M	Dukes'
I	TI	N0	M0	A
	T2	N0	M0	A
IIA	T3	N0	M0	B
IIB	T4	N0	M0	B
IIIA	TI–2	NI	M0	C
IIIB	T3–4	NI	M0	C
IIIC	Any T	N2	M0	C
IV	Any T	Any N	MI	D

Example: Hodgkin's lymphoma (Ann Arbor system)

■ Stage I: involvement of a single lymph node region, or of a single extra-lymphatic organ or site (I$_E$) NHL.

■ Stage II: involvement of ≥2 lymph node regions on the same side of the diaphragm or with involvement or with involvement of limited, contiguous extra-lymphatic organ or tissue (II$_E$).

■ Stage III: involvement of lymph node groups above and below the diaphragm, which may include the spleen (IIIS) or limited contiguous extra-lymphatic organs or site (IIIE).

■ Stage IV: multiple or disseminated foci of ≥1 extra-lymphatic organs or tissues with or without lymphatic involvement.

Cases are sub-classified according to the absence (A) or presence (B) of constitutional symptoms of significant fever, night sweats or unexplained weight loss exceeding 10% of normal body weight. Bulky disease comprising >10 cm or more than one-third widening of the mediastinum at T5 is denoted by the suffix X.

The Ann Arbor system is also employed to stage non-Hodgkin's lymphoma.

Grade

■ Pathological (histological) grade classifies tumours in terms of the degree of advancement or microscopic abnormality of the tumour cells.

■ Features considered by grade include overall growth and degree of invasion.

■ The degree of cellular differentiation is a description of how much the cells resemble the normal cells of the particular tissue type.

■ Grade is usually either a number from 1 to 4 (this can vary), or a general description of advancement (e.g. 'high' or 'low' grade).

■ Higher number = increasingly 'poor' differentiation (i.e. 'high' grade), i.e. a more advanced cancer.

■ Lower number = 'well' differentiated (i.e. 'low' grade), i.e. a less advanced cancer.

■ Certain tumours have their own grading systems. For example, prostate cancer is graded using the Gleason system (a 5-point score).

Standard grading system

■ GX = cannot be assessed

- G1 = well differentiated (low grade)
- G2 = moderately differentiated (intermediate grade)
- G3 = poorly differentiated (high grade)
- G4 = undifferentiated (high grade)

Example: Gleason grade
- Biopsies specimens graded (1–5 scale) according to differentiation of cells.

- The sum of the two highest grades = combined Gleason score, e.g. '3 + 4' or '7'.
- Low grade = score 2, 3 or 4.
- Intermediate grade = 5, 6 or 7.
- High grade = 8, 9 or 10.

Chapter 13
MICROBIOLOGY

Introduction

Infections are commonly encountered in almost all specialties of clinical medicine. The aim of this chapter is to provide an overview of the approach to their investigation and treatment. With an understanding of the basic principles underlying how this topic should be approached, it is possible to consider its application to individual specialities in more detail; further discussion of the specific specialty-based roles that microbiology can play is described in more detail within the various specialty chapters.

Topics covered
- Infection
- Systemic inflammatory response syndrome (SIRS)
- Approach to diagnosing infection
- Initial and further investigations
- Gram staining and identifying bacteria

- Imaging
- Antibiotic therapy
- Pyrexia of unknown origin
- Nosocomial infections
- Neutropaenic sepsis
- HIV/AIDS

Infection

Infection is defined as the invasion of the body's natural barriers by microscopic organisms – bacterial, fungal, viral or parasitic – which multiply to create symptoms.

Systemic inflammatory response syndrome (SIRS)

This is a process involving the release of various inflammatory mediators, including cytokines, free radicals and other vasoactive mediators. A diagnosis of SIRS requires two or more of the following:

- temperature: >38°C *or* <36°C
- pulse: >90 beats/min
- respiratory rate: >20 breaths/min *or* PCO_2 <4.3 kPa
- WCC: >12 × 10^9/L *or* <4 × 10^9/L *or* >10% immature (band) forms.

Sepsis

- SIRS in the presence of detectable infection.
- *NB:*
- bacteraemia alone is the asymptomatic presence of infective organisms, not necessarily sepsis.
- the term septicaemia was formerly used to imply multiplying bacteria in the bloodstream.

The hands-on guide to data interpretation. By S. Abraham, K. Kulkarni, R. Madhu and D. Provan. Published 2010 by Blackwell Publishing Ltd.

Severe sepsis

■ Sepsis with organ hypo-perfusion, e.g. hypoxia, oliguria, acidosis.

Septic shock

■ Severe sepsis with hypotension (systolic BP <90 mmHg).

■ Hypotension is often resistant to fluid resuscitation and vasopressor drugs.

Approach to diagnosing infection

■ Infection requires exposure to a pathogen.

■ This interacts with the host's immune system at a specific site.

■ This can then provoke local and systemic symptoms.

The approach to diagnosing an infection expands on the above areas.

Symptoms

■ Systemic: fever, night sweats, weight loss.

■ Focal: consider effects on each system (e.g. respiratory, genitourinary, etc.).

Exposure

■ Food (oral ingestion)
■ Occupational exposure
■ Travel: country, rural/urban areas, malaria prophylaxis, bites
■ Animal contact
■ Sexual contact
■ Intravenous drug use (IVDU)

Immunity

Predisposing factors for infection include the following.

■ Damaged barriers: lines, catheters, wounds, dental caries, *tinea*.

■ Diabetes mellitus (immunosuppressant and promotes pathogen growth).

■ Drugs (e.g. corticosteroids/ chemotherapy).

■ HIV risk factors present (have a lower threshold for investigating for both, the presence of HIV and any accompanying infection, if there are risk factors present).

Pyrexia (fever)

This is physiological resetting of the hypothalamic set point >37.5°C. Causes include:

■ infection
■ malignancy (e.g. lymphoma)
■ necrosis (e.g. myocardial infarction, MI)
■ venous thromboembolism (e.g. deep venous thrombosis, DVT)
■ connective tissue diseases (e.g. systemic lupus erythematosus, SLE)
■ drugs (e.g. beta-lactam fever).

Hyperpyrexia

This is loss of thermoregulation, causing temperature to rise excessively above the set point. Different sources quote different thresholds, but hyperpyrexia is usually defined as a temperature ≥41.0°C

Causes include:

■ infection/septicaemia
■ heat stroke (excessive sun exposure)
■ neuroleptic malignant syndrome (an adverse reaction to antipsychotic drugs)
■ malignant hyperthermia (anaesthetics)
■ drugs (e.g. ecstasy)
■ endocrine (e.g. thyrotoxic crisis)
■ neurological disorders (e.g. stroke).

Initial and further investigations

These aim to:
■ identify the causative organism
■ identify the site of infection
■ identify defects in host immunity predisposing to infection.

Baseline investigations

These include the following.
■ Urinalysis:
• nitrite *and* leucocyte esterase positive is specific for urinary tract infection, UTI; nitrite *or* leucocyte is sensitive but less specific.
■ Bloods:
• full blood count (FBC):
– neutrophils – rise in most bacterial infections
– lymphocytes – rise in most viral infections
– eosinophils – rise in most parasitic infections.
• C-reactive protein (CRP) or erythrocyte sedimentation rate (ESR) are broad inflammatory markers. They are particularly important if the patient is taking steroids (which can cause immunosuppression and elevate the white cell count (WCC) or if the patient is neutropaenic).
• glucose (diabetes mellitus predisposes to infection).
• urea and electrolytes/liver function tests/coagulation (can suggest end-organ dysfunction).
• blood cultures (should be taken before commencing antibiotic treatment).
■ chest X-ray (CXR).

Specialist microbiological tests

Specialist microbiological tests can be conducted on the following.

■ Blood.
■ Urine.
■ Stool.
■ Sputum.
■ Other fluid (e.g. cerebrospinal fluid (CSF), ascites, pleural fluid, samples from drains, etc.).
■ Skin swabs (these are non-sterile samples and are hence prone to contamination. They are more useful when looking for specific pathogens e.g. methicillin-resistant *Staphylooccus aureus* (MRSA) or herpes simplex virus (HSV)).
■ Biopsy samples (e.g. pleural biopsies in tuberculosis).

These specific microbiological investigations include the following.

Microscopy
■ Gram stain (blue = Gram-positive, red = Gram-negative organism).
■ Ziehl-Neelsen (ZN) stain – for acid-fast bacilli (tuberculosis).
■ Ova, cysts and parasites (OCP).
■ Electron microscopy (viruses).

Culture
■ Samples should ideally be taken before antibiotic therapy commences (otherwise the laboratory should be told what antibiotic been given, as this can affect culture and sensitivities).
■ Commonly used to identify many bacteria and fungi.
■ Once cultured, *in vitro* antimicrobial sensitivities can be used to determine which antibiotic agents the pathogen is susceptible to.

Serology
■ Antibody elevated in acute infection = IgM.
■ Sero-conversion = 4x rise in IgG titres.

Molecular techniques

■ Polymerase Chain Reaction (PCR) has a role (e.g. to determine viral load).

Histology

■ Effect of infection on tissues, e.g. granuloma (tuberculosis, TB) or inclusion bodies (cytomegalovirus, CMV).

Many of these techniques are specific but not sensitive for infection – repeat/multiple samples are often indicated (e.g. blood cultures).

Gram staining and identifying bacteria

■ Colony morphology and growth characteristics can give clues as to the causative organism.

■ Gram staining is a simple method for classifying many bacteria.

■ Gram-negative organisms have an additional layer of lipopolysaccharide (LPS) around their cell wall that stops staining. LPS (endotoxin) is partly

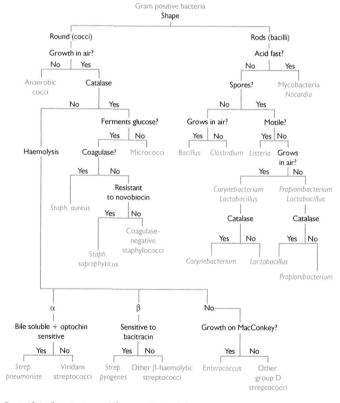

Figure 13.1: Gram-positive and Gram-negative bacteria

responsible for circulatory collapse in Gram-negative bacteraemia.

■ Bacterial shape can also aid identification. Gram-negative organisms tend to be rod-shaped (bacilli) whereas Gram-positives tend to be round (cocci).

■ Other means of identification include bacterial enzymes (e.g. staphylococcal coagulase), oxygen requirements, clustering, etc.

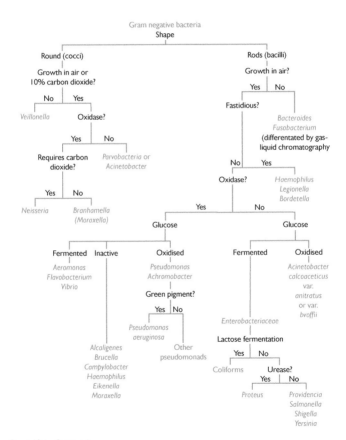

Figure 13.1: Continued

Imaging

The location of an infection using imaging techniques can aid management in two ways.

1 Determining treatment duration for specific infections (e.g. 6 weeks for endocarditis).

2 Increasing antimicrobial tissue availability by use of appropriate antibiotic (e.g. nitrofurantoin in UTI).

Additionally, imaging can be of use in localising inflammation or collections. Choice of modality depends on focal symptoms and signs, but commonly include:

■ echocardiogram (e.g. for endocarditis – ideally trans-oesophageal)

■ ultrasound (e.g. for collections)

■ CT (e.g. of chest, abdomen, pelvis, head)

■ MRI (e.g. for osteomyelitis, discitis).

Antibiotic therapy

■ Ideally, a clear microbiological diagnosis should be made before starting antibiotics to allow confident treatment with minimal side effects.

■ It can be helpful to consult a microbiologist early on to assist with management (e.g. helping to select appropriate investigations).

■ Inappropriate antibiotics may incompletely treat the infection, not treat it at all, have side effects, interfere with future samples (e.g. cultures) and, most importantly, can increase mortality.

■ Many of the above investigations take time – in most cases it is reasonable to wait for the results in order to use antibiotics that the organism is sensitive to.

■ However, if a patient is unwell (e.g. organ failure, shock, etc.) then empirical antibiotic therapy may be indicated, based on local guidelines.

■ Once an organism is subsequently identified, a microbiologist can advise further on how to modify treatment, if necessary.

Antibiotic sensitivity patterns

The table below shows a range of antibiotics and a broad indication of their ability in treating infections caused by specific organisms.

Organism	Penicillin	Amoxicillin	1st generation cephalosporin	3rd generation cephalosporin	Vancomycin	Erythromycin	Gentamicin	Tetracyclines	Clindamycin	Piperacillin	Chloramphenicol	Metronidazole
Gram +ve												
Group A Strep	✓	✓	✓	✓	✓	✓		✓	✓	✓		
Group B Strep	✓	✓	✓	✓	✓	✓		✓	✓	✓		
Enterococci (*synergy only)	✓	✓			✓		✓*			✓		
Listeria	✓	✓			✓							
Staph. aureus			✓	✓	✓	✓			✓	✓		
Strep. epidermidis					✓							
Strep. pneumonia	✓	✓	✓	✓	✓	✓				✓	✓	
Gram –ve												
E. coli			✓	✓			✓	✓		✓		
Enterobacter				✓			✓	✓		✓		
H. influenzae		✓		✓			✓	✓		✓	✓	
Klebsiella			✓	✓			✓			✓	✓	
N. meningitidis	✓	✓		✓				✓		✓		
Pseudomonas				✓			✓			✓		
Anaerobic												
Gut (+ = Gram-positives only)					✓+				+	✓		✓
Mouth	✓	✓								✓		✓

Bacterial resistance to antibiotic therapy

■ This occurs when an antibiotic loses its ability to effectively kill bacteria or to control their growth.

■ 'Survival of the fittest' evolutionary change drives bacterial resistance to antibiotic therapy; with a need to survive despite attack from antibiotics, it is the bacteria that are able to resist or counteract the effects of the drug that selectively survive and replicate over time.

■ Bacteria can acquire 'horizontal' genetic resistance through *spontaneous DNA mutation* (e.g. drug resistant tuberculosis), *transformation* (the uptake of DNA from another bacterium (e.g. penicillin-resistant gonorrhoea) or *conjugation* (the transfer of a plasmid, small circular DNA that can contain 'resistance' DNA, from one organism to another.

■ 'Vertical' spread when new generations of bacteria inherit resistance.

■ Inappropriate/overuse of antibiotic therapy contributes to the development of antibiotic resistance (e.g. use of antibiotics for viral infections).

Pyrexia of unknown origin (PUO)

This is defined as undiagnosed fever >38.3°C after 3 weeks' investigation, which includes 1 week in hospital.

Investigation should be as for all infections (see above). In particular, consider the following.

■ Basic observations (e.g. temperature, pulse, etc.; see Chapter 16 for more details)

■ Bedside tests (electrocardiogram, urinalysis)

■ Basic bloods (including full blood count, inflammatory markers, renal/liver function)

■ Extended cultures (including blood, urine, etc.)

■ Imaging (e.g. CXR, CT of abdomen and pelvis)

■ Echocardiography (initially trans-thoracic)

■ Bone marrow aspirate

■ Autoantibody screen

Empirical treatment may be given in certain cases.

■ Anti-tuberculous treatment if high risk

■ Steroids if elderly (e.g. ?giant cell arteritis)

Nosocomial infections

■ These are 'hospital-acquired' infections, i.e. those that occur ≥48 h post-admission or within 30 days of discharge).

■ Hospitalised patients at particular risk, include those with:

• co-morbid illness

• exposure to virulent pathogens

• prior use of antibiotics

• procedures (e.g. surgery, lines, catheters, etc.).

Infections to consider

Staphylococcal infections

■ Organisms such as *S. aureus* enter the bloodstream via lines; initial steps should therefore involve checking line-insertion sites and the removal of any that appear infected/inflamed or are unused (e.g. peripheral venous cannulae, central lines).

■ Classically disseminates causing multi-focal collections.

■ Bacteraemia (presence of organism in the bloodstream) requires 2 weeks' treatment (intravenous therapy).

■ Sepsis requires at least 6 weeks' treatment.

■ MRSA needs a less effective and potentially more toxic antibiotic (e.g. vancomycin) that is less convenient to administer regularly.

NB: For more detailed definitions of these terms, see Chapter 16.

Gram-negative sepsis

■ The source of these infections is usually from the urine or gastrointestinal tract.

■ The LPS causes a systemic inflammatory reaction (shock, acute respiratory distress syndrome, ARDS).

Clostridium difficile (C. diff)

■ Diagnosed by detection of toxins A AND B in the faeces of a symptomatic patient.

■ Disease can be classified from mild to life threatening:

• mild disease = ≤3 episodes of diarrhoea (Type 5–7, Bristol Stool chart) per 24-h period and a normal WCC

• moderate disease = 3–5 episodes of diarrhoea (Type 5–7, Bristol Stool chart) per 24h period and a raised WCC, but still less than 20,000/mm³ (20 × 10⁹/L)

• severe disease = number of episodes of diarrhoea (Type 5–7, Bristol Stool chart) is considered to be a less reliable indicator of severe disease. WCC >20,000 (20 × 10⁹/L) or temperature >38.5°C or acute rising serum creatinine (e.g. >50% increase above baseline) or

evidence of severe colitis (abdominal or radiological signs)

• complicated disease = hypotension, partial ileus or CT evidence of severe disease

• life threatening disease = complete ileus or toxic megacolon.

■ Infection often follows the use of broad-spectrum antibiotics such as the cefalosporins, ciprofloxacin or clindamycin.

■ Three stool samples should be sent for toxin assay (CDT). Note that this can stay positive for up to 4 weeks after treatment.

■ Treatment involves oral antibiotics (such as vancomycin, metronidazole). *NB:* Metronidazole can be given IV if needed.

Neutropaenic sepsis

■ Sepsis in the presence of low neutrophil count (<1.0 × 10⁹/L), leading to an increased susceptibility to infection.

■ The risk of infection is greater the faster the rate of decline of the neutrophil count and the longer the duration of neutropaenia (especially if neutropaenia lasts for >10 days).

■ For example, patients on cytotoxic chemotherapy often fail to produce neutrophils due to bone marrow suppression.

■ This leaves them at risk of overwhelming sepsis, often with little warning.

■ It is important to treat these patients quickly (before they look unwell) with broad-spectrum such as meropenem.

HIV/AIDS

■ A full account of HIV medicine is beyond the scope of this book.

■ If a patient with HIV has a low CD4 cell count (<200 cells/mm³ blood) then they are at risk of opportunistic infections and need specialist investigation and treatment.

■ Patients become more susceptible to a different range of infections, depending on the CD4 count. For example:

• 200–500 cells/mm³: pneumonia, tuberculosis, fungal infections

• <200 cells/mm³: *Pneumocystis carinii* pneumonia (PCP) and fungal infections

• <50 cells/mm³: cytomegalovirus (CMV) and *Mycobacterium avium* complex (MAC) infection.

■ Another important laboratory measure is HIV viral load, a measurement of HIV nucleic acid (RNA), used as a measure of the degree of replication activity of the virus. Numbers vary depending on the assay used, but during treatment and monitoring a high viral load can be between 5,000 and 10,000 copies/mL. Initial, untreated viral loads can be over 1,000,000 copies/mL. A low viral load is usually between 40 and 500 copies/mL.

■ It is clear that many new cases of HIV have often been hospitalised with infections prior to their diagnosis. It is becoming increasingly accepted that patients hospitalised for infectious diseases without a clear predisposition (e.g. extremes of age, co-morbidity) should be offered an HIV test.

■ An HIV test should always be preceded by appropriate counselling to ensure that the patient is fully aware of what the test involves, as well as the consequences of a positive result.

Chapter 14
GENETICS

Introduction

Many disease processes have a genetic component. However, a basic understanding of genetics is lacking as it is an undertaught field. With the advent of increased genetic screening tools (e.g. genetic screening to estimate a patient's likely response to a particular drug), the importance/relevance of genetics in clinical medicine is likely to increase. This chapter considers the basics of the various patterns of Mendelian inheritance and discusses some more commonly encountered chromosomal abnormalities.

Topics covered
■ Patterns of inheritance
■ Chromosomal abnormalities

Patterns of inheritance

■ Mendelian inheritance usually takes either an 'autosomal' form (related to chromosomes 1–22) or a 'sex-linked' form (related to chromosomes X or Y).
■ Other modes of inheritance include mitochondrial (these have their own DNA) and genetic imprinting (genes expressed only if either paternal or maternal, e.g. Prader-Willi syndrome).

■ A change in genetic code (genotype) can be clinically expressed in different ways (phenotypes).
■ Variable inheritance patterns can be present. These include 'non-penetrance' (genotypic disease but no phenotypic features) or 'anticipation' (symptomatically worse disease as generations progress).
■ Genotype 'errors' can not only be inherited, but can also be formed as new mutations (in previously normal lineage).
■ Looking at the pattern of disease progression through a family tree can help determine the type of inheritance.

The hands-on guide to data interpretation. By S. Abraham, K. Kulkarni, R. Madhu and D. Provan. Published 2010 by Blackwell Publishing Ltd.

Family tree

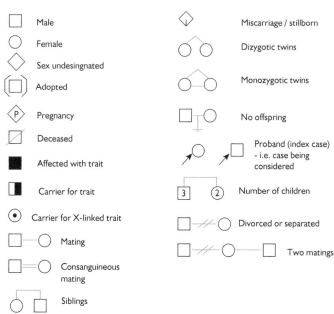

□ Male	◇ Miscarriage / stillborn
○ Female	○╱╲○ Dizygotic twins
◇ Sex undesignated	○╱╲○ Monozygotic twins
▢ Adopted	□┬○ No offspring
◇ P Pregnancy	
◇ Deceased	↗○ ↗□ Proband (index case) - i.e. case being considered
■ Affected with trait	
◨ Carrier for trait	③ ② Number of children
⊙ Carrier for X-linked trait	□─//─○ Divorced or separated
□──○ Mating	□─//─○──□ Two matings
□══○ Consanguineous mating	
○ □ Siblings	

Figure 14.1: Commonly used symbols in family trees

Autosomal recessive (AR)

For example cystic fibrosis, sickle cell disease, Tay-Sachs, thalassaemia, Wilson's disease, haemochromatosis, phenylketonuria, Friedreich's ataxia.
With one parent a carrier:
■ 50% of offspring will be carriers
■ males and females are equally susceptible.
With both parents carriers:
■ 50% of offspring will be carriers
■ 25% of offspring will be affected
■ 25% of offspring will be normal
■ males and females are equally susceptible.

With one parent affected:
■ 100% of offspring will be carriers
■ males and females are equally susceptible.

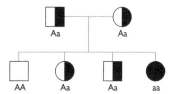

Figure 14.2: Autosomal recessive inheritance

Autosomal dominant (AD)

For example, adult polycystic kidney disease, neurofibromatosis, Marfan's syndrome, Ehler-Danlos syndrome, osteogenesis imperfecta, myotonic dystrophy, familial hypercholesterolaemia, Huntington's disease.

With one parent affected:

■ 50% chance of offspring being affected, 50% chance of normal offspring

■ males and females are equally affected.

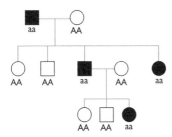

Figure 14.3: Autosomal dominant inheritance

Sex-linked (X-linked recessive)

For example, haemophilia A and B, Duchenne muscular dystrophy, Becker's muscular dystrophy, fragile X syndrome.

With a carrier mother:

■ 50% of males will be affected

■ 50% of females will be carriers

■ 50% of offspring will be normal

■ only males are affected.

With an affected father (normal mother):

■ 100% of males will be normal

■ 100% of females will be carriers

■ 0% of male and female offspring will be affected.

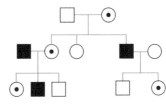

Figure 14.4: X-linked recessive inheritance

Sex-linked (X-linked dominant)

For example, Vitamin D-resistant rickets.

With an affected mother:

■ 50% of male offspring will be affected

■ 50% of female offspring will be affected.

With an affected father:

■ 100% of male offspring will be normal

■ 100% of female offspring will be affected.

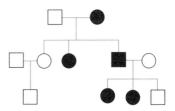

Figure 14.5: X-linked dominant inheritance

Mitochondrial

For example, Leber's hereditary optic neuropathy.

■ Mitochondrial DNA is inherited from maternal genes only.

■ Affected males do not pass on the condition to their offspring.

■ Affected females can pass on the condition to their offspring.
■ Both males and females are affected.

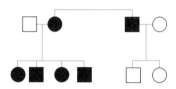

Figure 14.6: Mitochondrial inheritance

Chromosomal abnormalities

■ Autosomal chromosomes (1–22) are present as two identical copies (pairs), with a single pair of sex chromosomes).

■ This is the karyotype (i.e. the total complement of chromosomes for a species).

■ Common karyotype abnormalities involving specific chromosomes, include:

• 46 XX / 46 XY: normal female/male
• 47 XXY: Klinefelter's syndrome
• 47 XXX: triple-X syndrome
• 47 XYY: males, increased incidence of personality problems (e.g. aggressive behaviour).

Mutations

Individual chromosomes can undergo mutations. Examples of conditions include:

■ cystic fibrosis (chromosome 7 – CFTR, cystic fibrosis transmembrane regulator)
■ haemochromatosis (chromosome 6 – HFE gene).

Trisomies

These involve the presence of three chromosomes, instead of the usual pair. Conditions include:

■ 13: Patau syndrome
■ 18: Edwards' syndrome
■ 21: Down syndrome.

Chapter 15
IMAGING

Introduction

With the increased reliance on imaging in clinical practice, a thorough discussion of data interpretation in radiology could occupy a vast textbook on its own. This chapter therefore intends to be more of an *aide mémoire* – a guide to help you learn the key facts about some of the more commonly encountered imaging investigations. The key is to practise interpreting and presenting real cases – particularly for the common pathologies. Always remember to compare images with previous ones, and do not forget to interpret any findings in the clinical context. Isolated imaging is of limited value. Always look, and then keep looking for more. Combined with a set framework for looking through images (e.g. X-rays), this is of great value, as it will ensure that you are thorough with your interpretation.

Topics covered
■ The basics
■ Chest X-ray interpretation
■ Abdominal X-ray interpretation
■ Ultrasound
■ Echocardiography
■ Computed tomography (CT)

■ Magnetic resonance imaging (MRI)
■ Nuclear imaging
■ Contrast studies
■ Bone density imaging
■ Radiation doses
■ Presenting imaging findings
■ Tips on making radiology requests

The basics

There are a number of general rules for looking at and interpreting all imaging investigations.
■ When interpreting X-rays, it is important to ensure you are thorough and work through the image using a set system. When reviewing imaging studies, make sure you are placed in the correct atmosphere, e.g. radiologists report films from within darkened rooms to remove light contamination from other sources,

thereby improving the chance of detecting subtle abnormalities.
■ Most hospitals that have implemented hospital-wide picture archiving and communication systems (PACS) employ two systems to deliver the images. One deals with higher quality (DICOM) images (for the higher quality monitors used by the radiologists to report films). The second utilises lower quality (usually JPEG) images to supply ward- or clinic-based lower quality monitors (for clinicians to review).

The hands-on guide to data interpretation. By S. Abraham, K. Kulkarni, R. Madhu and D. Provan. Published 2010 by Blackwell Publishing Ltd.

■ If you have a printed film, use a light box to view it. A bright light should be used for reviewing any areas of uncertainty.

■ If you are looking at an X-ray on a PC monitor, use the brightness and contrast adjustments to bring out more detail. Ward-based PACS software will have the ability to adjust these, as well as zoom, magnify and measure on the image. Make sure you learn how to use the systems well to get the most out of them.

■ Try to look at any of the previous imaging, for comparison. This will help you determine whether any findings are acute or chronic. If the imaging is not available, try to read the previous reports for comparison. The best is to do both.

■ If you find one abnormality, make sure you keep looking for more – it can be tempting to stop there and you may miss other signs.

■ Always check the left and right side markers first.

The key is practice – look at as many films as possible and read the report afterwards to see if you have missed any features. Presenting films to seniors can be a very helpful way of practising how would present an X-ray during an exam. Ensure that you mention all of the key positive and negative findings.

Chest X-ray (CXR) interpretation

■ This is the most commonly performed radiological examination, hence the most important one to understand.

■ This section is intended to be an aide mémoire that you can use to remind yourself of the key stages of CXR interpretation.

Check the technical details
■ Patient details: name, DOB, hospital number
■ Date of X-ray
■ Direction of X-ray beam (posteroanterior (PA), anteroposterior (AP), lateral, etc.)
■ Position of patient (supine, erect, semi-erect)
■ Orientation (which is left and right?)
■ Adequate penetration? (minimal vessels should be visible in the outer parts of the lungs and the intervertebral discs should just be visible through the middle of the cardiac shadow)
■ Adequate inspiration? (in full inspiration, 6–7 anterior ribs or 10–11 posterior ribs should be visible)
■ Any rotation? (equal distance between the medial end of both clavicles and the spinous processes?)
• inequality in the left and right distances could mean there is rotation: this occurs to the side of the larger distance (e.g. if the distance is larger on the right compared with the left, then the patient is rotated to the right)
• this is important in order to account for the difference in transradiancy of the hemithoraces

Look at the cardiac shadow
(Figure 15.1)

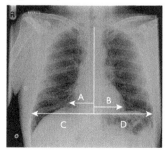

Figure 15.1: Normal male chest X-ray

■ Size:
• cardiac transverse diameter = A + B = <15.5 cm (male), <15.0 cm (female)
• cardiothoracic ratio = (A + B) / (C + D) = <0.5.

■ Shape (look for any localised or global abnormal dilatation).
■ Calcification (e.g. of valves).
■ Position (one-third to right of midline, two-thirds to left of midline).

Look at the rest of the mediastinum (Figure 15.2)

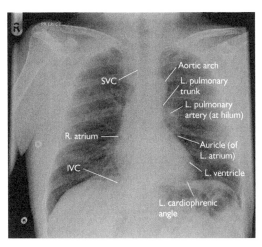

Figure 15.2: Normal male chest X-ray

■ Outline/borders – from top to bottom:
• right: brachiocephalic vein, superior vena cava (SVC), right atrium, inferior vena cava (IVC)
• left: left pulmonary artery, left atrial appendage, left ventricle
• aorta and aortic contour – look for calcification, dilatation or aneurysm formation
• mediastinal widening: note that the mediastinum will look widened on an AP film compared to a PA film, and also when the patient is supine compared to erect.

Look at the position of the hila
■ In mid-axillary line:
• right: 6th rib
• left: up to 2.5 cm higher.

Look at the lung fields
■ Size (assess based on number of visible ribs as above):
• increased: chronic onstructive pulmonary disease (COPD) (bilateral)
• decreased: fibrosis (bilateral), lobar collapse (localised loss of volume).
■ Transradiancy, for example:
• COPD: blacker and hyperinflated

- lobar pneumonia: localised consolidation (borders follow edges of lobe and fissures), air bronchograms
- collapse: deviated fissures:
  - left upper lobe: hazy outline to most of left lung field
  - left lower lobe: 'sail' sign behind left heart border
  - right upper lobe: raised horizontal fissure, wedge shaped opacity at top of right lung field
  - right middle lobe: blurred right heart border
  - right lower lobe: blurred right diaphragm border.

■ Fissures in correct places? (e.g. horizontal fissure).

■ Consolidation (shadowing of the air spaces):

- is it local or generalised?
- air bronchograms (suggest consolidation)
- upper lobe diversion, Kerley-B lines and enlarged heart (pulmonary oedema)
- 'white-out' of entire lung field (acute respiratory distress syndrome (ARDS) or non-cardiogenic pulmonary oedema)
- localised opacity +/− air fluid levels or hilar lymphadeopathy or collapse (malignancy, tuberculosis (TB), abscess)
- fine reticulo-nodular shadowing/ ground-glass shadowing/honeycombing (fibrosis).

Fibrosis

The mnemonics 'ESCHART' and 'RASCO' can be used to help remember the causes of pulmonary fibrosis.

Upper (apical) fibrosis	Lower (basal) fibrosis
Extrinsic allergic alveolitis	**R**heumatoid arthritis
Sarcoidosis	**A**sbestosis
Cystic fibrosis (can be lower lobe too)	**S**cleroderma
Histiocytosis X	**C**ryptogenic fibrosing alveolitis (aka idiopathic pulmonary fibrosis)
Allergic bronchopulmonary aspergillosis, ankylosing spondylitis	**O**ther (drugs: bleomycin, nitrofurantoin, amiodarone)
Radiotherapy	
TB	

Look at the pleural spaces

■ Pleural effusion: basal curved opacity with a meniscus at either end, unless the X-ray is performed supine, when a pleural effusion may appear as just diffusely increased opacity in the affected lung. (Remember pleural effusion can contain serous fluid or blood – it is important to know the history as you can't differentiate between them on the X-ray.)

■ Pneumothorax (unilateral blackening, fewer visible vessels, white pleural outline visible, deviated trachea or shifted mediastinal contents in tension pneumothorax – a medical emergency).

■ Hydropneumothorax: this will have an air–fluid level; the inferior fluid component will have a totally flat upper border with no meniscus. The superior air-containing component will be as a pneumothorax.

■ Note the differences between X-rays taken when the patient is erect and when they are supine.

Look at the bones

■ Any lesions:
• lytic/sclerotic lesions (metastasis)
• fractures (remember the history).
■ Notching (coarctation of the aorta).

Look at the surrounding soft tissues

■ Under the diaphragm (for pneumoperitoneum).

■ Breasts:
• symmetrical (mastectomy)
• any masses or abnormal calcification?
■ Other structures/equipment:
• pacemaker
• ECG lead
• venous access lines (look for their position; which access route has been used, such as via the right internal jugular vein; where the tip is; and possibly also for a post-insertion pneumothorax).

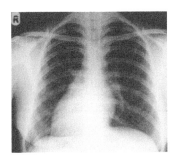

Figure 15.3: Dextrocardia

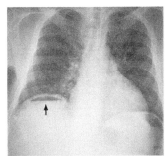

Figure 15.5: Pneumoperitoneum

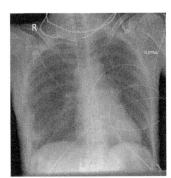

Figure 15.4: Rib fractures, with flail segment

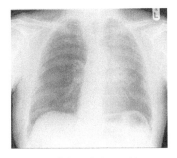

Figure 15.6: Collapse of left upper lobe

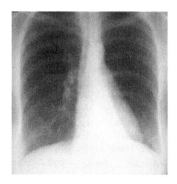

Figure 15.7: Collapse of left lower lobe

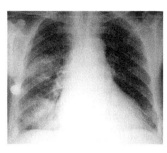

Figure 15.10: Collapse of right lower lobe

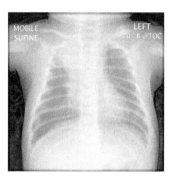

Figure 15.8: Collapse of right upper lobe

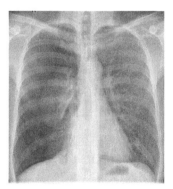

Figure 15.11: Simple pneumothorax

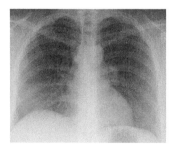

Figure 15.9: Collapse of right middle lobe

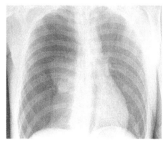

Figure 15.12: Tension pneumothorax

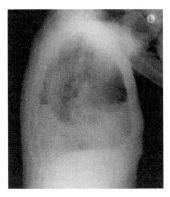

Figure 15.13: Pleural effusion, lateral view

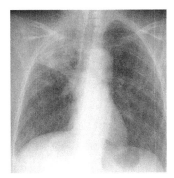

Figure 15.16: Tuberculosis

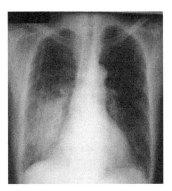

Figure 15.14: Pneumonia consolidation

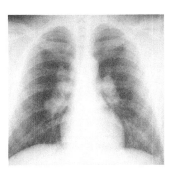

Figure 15.17: Sarcoid

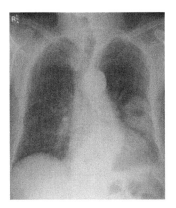

Figure 15.15: Lung abscess

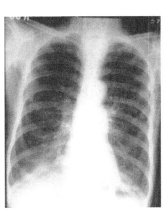

Figure 15.18: Fibrosis

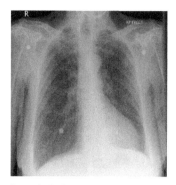

Figure 15.19: Chronic obstructive pulmonary disease

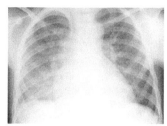

Figure 15.21: Congestive heart failure and cardiomegaly

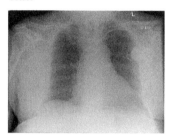

Figure 15.20: Pacemaker

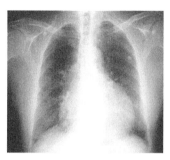

Figure 15.22: Pericardial effusion

Abdominal X-ray (AXR) interpretation

The basic structure of AXR interpretation is similar to the section above.

Check the technical details
- Patient details: name, DOB, hospital number
- Date of X-ray
- Projection (PA, AP, lateral, oblique, etc.)
- Patient position (should preferably be supine)
- Orientation (which is left and right?)

Look at the large and small bowel patterns
Small bowel
- Valvulae conniventae (go all the way around the bowel circumference)
- Narrow (maximum 3.5 cm proximally, 2.5 cm distally)
- No fluid level should be visible in a supine AXR (although in an erect film, up to five visible fluid levels is usually considered normal)
- Mainly located in the centre of the film

Large bowel
- Haustra (only go partially around bowel circumference)

- Can contain faeces
- Wider (maximum 6 cm at transverse colon or 9 cm at caecum)
- Mainly located in the periphery of the film

Sentinel loops of bowel
- Single, usually central loop of dilated bowel (small or large)
- Associated with: acute abdomen (acute pancreatitis/cholecystitis/appendicitis, etc.)

Look for abnormal gas patterns
- Pneumoperitoneum (although this better visualised on an erect chest X-ray).
- Gas in the bowel wall:
- infections (e.g. pneumatosis)
- premature neonates (necrotising enterocolitis)
- ischaemia and bowel necrosis.
- Rigler's sign:
- gas either side of the bowel wall – free intraperitoneal air
- may be normal post-laparotomy and pelvic surgery due to insufflation of abdominal cavity with gas.
- Retroperitoneal gas:
- e.g. colonic perforation or necrotising acute pancreatitis.
- Gas in the biliary tree:
- gallstone ileus with cholecystoenteric fistula
- post-ERCP/sphincterotomy/biliary drainage.
- Gas in the urinary tract:
- colovesical fistula (secondary to diverticular disease, Crohn's disease (IBD), colonic malignancy, etc.).
- Gas-forming infections (although these tend to from abscesses, they can also be a cause of a number of the above, e.g. gas in the gallbladder or urinary tract – particularly in certain patients such as those with diabetes mellitus). These can also be the cause of gas in the abdominal wall.

Look for abnormal calcification
- Calculi: gallstones, urinary tract stones (including staghorn, renal, ureteric and bladder calculi)
- Viscera: gall bladder, pancreas (chronic pancreatitis)
- Vascular: aortic aneurysms
- Malignancy: can appear as abnormal calcification

Look for other structures and viscera
Viscera
Organs are usually delineated by interfaces between differing densities, e.g. between fat and air around the bowel, or calcification (see above). Aside from those already discussed, you may occasionally see other organs, particularly when they are enlarged, e.g. a larger liver or kidney shadows.

Retroperitoneal
Loss of the psoas outlines, although normal in 20% of the population, may suggest masses or haematomas in the retroperitoneal space.

Bones
Check for the integrity of the vertebrae, as well as that of other bones including the pelvis and the femur and ribs (if visible).

Herniae
Look at the femoral and inguinal hernial sites, for the presence of abnormal bowel loops. If there are bowel loops in those sites, then there may be a hernia containing either small or large bowel; this may incarcerate and cause bowel obstruction.

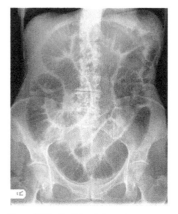

Figure 15.23: Small bowel obstruction

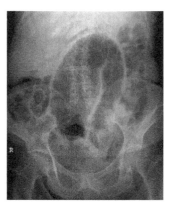

Figure 15.25: Sigmoid volvulus

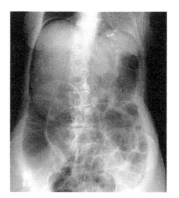

Figure 15.24: Large bowel obstruction

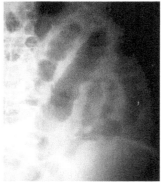

Figure 15.26: Crohn's disease and mucosal oedema (thumb printing)

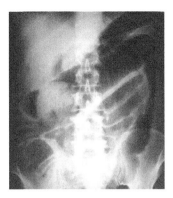

Figure 15.27: Toxic megacolon

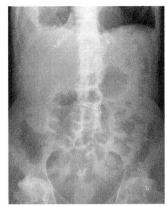

Figure 15.28: Gallstones and mucosal oedema (thumb printing)

Ultrasound

■ Ultrasonography uses high-frequency sound waves (2–10 MHz) that are varyingly reflected by different tissues.

■ This non-invasive test has a number of diagnostic and therapeutic uses, for example measuring the dimensions of blood vessels (e.g. aorta, carotid artery), guiding drainage and biopsy procedures, and physiotherapy.

■ However, this technique is not ideal for assessing structures consisting of air or bone. Ultrasound waves poorly penetrate bone and are reflected by gas (hence fail to pass through). This therefore limits its use, for example when requiring visualisation of the bowel or structures the other side of the air (i.e. the other side of the bowel).

■ Diagnostic ultrasound has no contraindications. However, other forms/uses of ultrasound (such as Doppler or therapeutic ultrasound use in physiotherapy) have the potential to cause temperature rises (although this would probably require imaging for hours at a time). These are theoretically potentially harmful to foetal development and should be used with caution.

Common investigative uses

Abdominal imaging

■ Commonly used for investigating a number of conditions, including biliary disease (gallstones), renal disease, bleeds (e.g. focused ultrasound in splenic injury) and aortic dimensions (normal diameter considered to be approximately 3 cm and of 'concern' when >5.5 cm).

Obstetric imaging

■ Including determining the age and sex of the foetus, screening for abnormalities, observing foetal movement and physiological status (heart rate, respiration) as well as assessing foetal growth.

Trans-vaginal (women) and transrectal ultrasound (TRUS, men)

■ Detection of pelvic pathology (e.g. ovarian and prostate cancer, respectively).

■ Assessment of prostate size.

NB: TRUS is not very sensitive for prostate tumour detection but random biopsies are possible and still the current standard.

Doppler and duplex imaging

■ Uses the Doppler effect to calculate frequency shifts and subsequently flow velocity and direction.

■ The flow, for example in blood vessels, can either be heard as an audio wave or displayed on screen. 3–7 MHz are generally used for peripheral vascular imaging (higher frequencies provide better resolution and more detail, but have less depth of penetration).

■ Duplex imaging takes things further by allowing the display of colour Doppler images, with different colours representing different velocities. Different colours are assigned to depict flow towards or away from the ultrasound probe.

Cardiac echosonography

■ To observe cardiac contraction and determine left ventricular ejection fraction.

■ Normal ejection fraction is usually defined as ≥55%.

Transoesophageal echo (TOE)

■ Utilises an endoscope-like device with an ultrasound probe at its tip.

■ Often used to investigate aortic dissection, prosthetic valve dysfunction and infective endocarditis.

■ Requires patient sedation.

High intensity focused ultrasound (HIFU)

■ A new technique employing ultrasound with lower frequencies but higher energies than conventional ultrasound.

■ Used for treating benign and malignant tumours (e.g. prostate cancer).

Extracorporeal shock wave lithotripsy (ESWL)

■ Uses a powerful focused ultrasound source to break up calculi.

Echocardiography

■ It is useful to understand the basics of this imaging modality, often termed 'cardiac echo', so that you can understand routine trasthoracic echocardiogram reports.

■ Here are some general points to note.

Pulmonary artery pressure	Estimate pressure >35 mmHg = hypertension
Chamber dimensions	L atrium = 4.5 diameter, L ventricle = 5.5 cm diameter
Interventricular septum dimension	<1.2 cm
Left ventricular function (ejection fraction) – i.e. fraction of blood expelled in each systole	>55%
Valves	■ Stenosis categories: mild, moderate severe ■ Pressure gradients and valve areas can quantify severity
Other features to note	■ Vegetations (endocarditis) ■ Tumours (e.g. atrial myxoma) ■ Thrombi (e.g. in AF) ■ Pericardial effusions

NB: Numbers quoted are general reference values, and may vary between normal, healthy individuals.

More recent updates to this established technique include three-dimensional echo. This allows more detailed imaging of the anatomical structure of the heart and can be helpful in the diagnosis of valvular and myocardial disease.

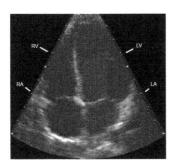

Figure 15.29: Echocardiogram

Computed tomography (CT)

■ This involves the generation of a three-dimensional image, effectively from the collection of a series of high-resolution two-dimensional X-ray image slices taken around a single axis of rotation.

■ The radiointensity of the imaged tissues is calculated using the Hounsfield scale, for example with air being −1,000 Hounsfield units (HU) and bone being >400 HU. The difference in radiointensity provides the ability to differentiate and delineate different tissues.

■ By technique known as 'windowing', the calculated Hounsfield units are used to form an image. Different scanners can produce images with different degrees of resolution, and different image processing modalities utilise different protocols to calculate different ranges of Hounsfield units.

■ There are a number of different image acquisition methods, including spiral/helical CT and multi-slice CT, etc. These all have their own image gathering properties and resolutions, hence are suited to different applications.

■ Contrast-enhanced CT can utilise intravenous contrast agents (usually iodine containing), oral contrast agents (iodine or barium containing, water or various special oral agents) or a combination of both to help visualise certain tissue structures. The three key planes in which CTs can be viewed are (Figure 15.31):

• transverse or axial (a horizontal slice through the body)

• coronal (like a coronation crown)

• sagittal (like being stabbed with a sword).

■ CT imaging plays a key role in the diagnosis of a number of conditions, including:

• *neurological*: e.g. cerebrovascular accidents (CVA, with a high sensitivity for detecting bleeds routinely used in the acute phase to distinguish ischaemic from haemorrhagic strokes)

• *respiratory*: e.g. pulmonary embolus (CT pulmonary angiogram, CTPA, allows the embolus to be visualised), interstitial lung disease

• *vascular*: e.g. aortic dissection or aneurism rupture, arterial stenosis or occlusion

• *oncology*: malignancy (primary staging and follow-up)

• *abdominal*: CT is an important test in the investigation of abdominal pain, inflammatory bowel disease and bowel obstruction. CT colonography can be used instead of barium enema to study the colon

• *urinary tract*: CT urogram (CTU) is increasingly replacing intravenous urogram (IVU) for the imaging of urinary tract obstruction caused by pathologies such as calculi

• *cardiac*: to study cardiac morphology, function, and to assess the coronary arteries for coronary heart disease.

■ CT can also play a role in more therapeutic aspects of management, for example as the imaging modality of choice in radiologically guided invasive procedures such as CT-guided biopsies.

■ Faster speed and lower relative cost are two of the advantages of CT over MRI imaging. Furthermore, CT has improved spatial resolution over MRI (the ability to distinguish two structures a particular distance apart, as distinct entities).

■ However, CT does use ionising radiation. A CT of the chest has the equivalent radiation dose of 400 chest X-rays, or 3 years' natural background radiation. Careful clinical consideration needs to be taken before requesting CT and other high radiation dose imaging investigations on children and pregnant women.

■ Iodinated contrast agents used intravenously are known to have nephrotoxic effects, especially in patients with already poor renal function. They can also cause metabolic problems for patients taking metformin. Most hospitals already have a local policy with regard to these situations – it is important to know your local hospital policy.

NB: More detail about these specialist types of MRI can be found in the respective specialty chapters.

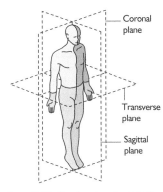

Figure 15.30: Three key planes in which CTs can be viewed

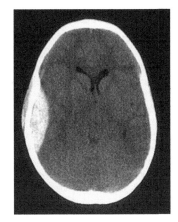

Figure 15.32: Extradural haemorrhage

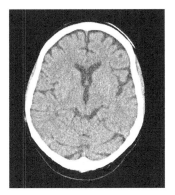

Figure 15.31: Normal head CT

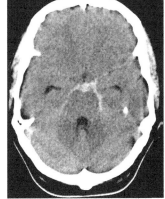

Figure 15.33: Subarachnoid haemorrhage

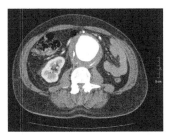

Figure 15.34: Abdominal aortic aneurysm

Magnetic resonance imaging (MRI)

■ MRI imaging utilises the relaxation properties of excited hydrogen nuclei in water and lipids.

■ When placed in a magnetic field, hydrogen atoms (protons) spin, aligning themselves parallel to the magnetic field. A radiofrequency pulse is then sent to 'knock' the hydrogen nuclei 'off balance'. When this pulse is stopped, the hydrogen nuclei will 'relax' back to the alignment they were in, parallel to the magnetic field. In doing so, the hydrogen nuclei release energy as radiofrequency waves, which is listened for. The varying concentration and state of hydrogen nuclei in different tissues (e.g. fat, muscle, bone) will alter the speed at which individual and groups of hydrogen nuclei relax, thereby varying the radiofrequency energy that is released. This allows differentiation between tissue types.

■ A key advantage that MRI has over CT, is the fact that it does not utilise ionising radiation. This makes it safer, particularly in certain patient groups (e.g. pregnant women or those requiring repeated imaging). Furthermore, MRI has improved contrast resolution than CT (the ability to distinguish two tissues that have broadly similar but non-identical appearances).

■ However, MRI does have lower spatial resolution than CT. MRI imaging takes longer to perform than CT and involves the patient lying still in a relatively small tunnel during that time; the scanner is also very noisy. It is therefore potentially unsuitable for those who suffer from claustrophobia, cannot lie motionless for the examination, or patients who need to be monitored closely during the examination.

■ Because high-intensity magnetic fields are used, MRI cannot be performed on patients who have implanted medical devices whose function would be disturbed by the magnetic field, e.g. cardiac pacemakers. Other implants (e.g. hip prostheses) may not prevent MRI being performed if they have been in for a sufficiently long time. However, they may cause artefacts on the MRI images, which can compromise reporting quality. It is important to put all the details of any implanted devices (e.g. coronary stents), including the type, brand and model of device, on the request so that the radiology department can decide in advance if MRI imaging can be performed on that particular patient.

■ MRI is highly sensitive for visualising soft tissues, and images can be contrast-enhanced (e.g. using gadolinium) to help localise pathological from normal tissues.

■ There are two commonly used image weightings:
• T1-weighting
• T2-weighting: reversed contrast, with 'water appearing white'.

■ There are also several different specific or specialised MRI types, such as diffusion-weighted images (useful in neurological imaging, e.g. of ischaemic tissue), or magnetic resonance spectroscopy (useful for visualising metabolic activity).

■ The contrast agents used in MRI are gadolinium chelates. These are in themselves nephrotoxic, and have to be used with care in patients with poor renal function (can cause renal failure in the short term, and fibrosis in the long term).

Differences between T1- and T2-weighted images

	T1	T2
Overall	Better for anatomical detail (e.g. differences between solid and cystic structures)	Better for pathological changes
Basic principle	Measures how protons align relative to external magnetic field	Measures how protons align relative to one another
Bone (cortex)	Light grey	Dark – black
White matter	White/light grey	Dark grey
Grey matter	Grey	Light grey
Water (e.g. oedema, vitreous, CSF)	Dark – black	Bright – light grey/ white ('**W**ater = **W**hite')
Fat (lipid)	Bright – white	Light grey
Muscle	Grey	Grey
Air	Dark – black	Dark – black
Blood (haematoma)	Sub-acute bleed: bright rim with core of varying intensity	Acute bleed: bright rim with dark core Chronic/old bleed: dark rim

T1:

T2:

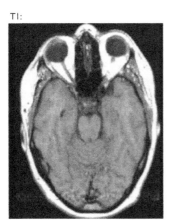 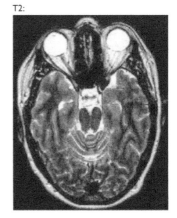

Figure 15.35: T1 versus T2

MRI applications/techniques

Specific MRI applications/techniques include the following.

■ Cardiac MRI and magnetic resonance angiography (MRA):

• these are relatively new techniques that can provide enhanced imaging of the heart and vessels, respectively

• cardiac MRI allows detailed visualisation of the myocardium during contraction and can therefore be used in the diagnosis of congenital heart disease, disorders of the heart muscle and in valvular pathologies

• MRA is a non-invasive technique for visualising the coronary blood vessels.

■ Magnetic resonance venography (MRV):

• this is a recently developed technique that is of use in imaging venous disease, e.g. deep venous thrombosis.

■ Functional MRI (fMRI):

• this can be used to measure functional cardiac activity, e.g. neural activity of different brain regions, based on varying degrees of oxygen consumption.

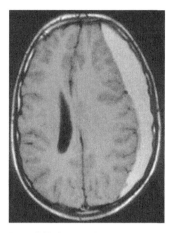

Figure 15.37: Subdural bleed

Nuclear imaging

■ Otherwise known as 'radionuclide radiology' or 'nuclear imaging'.

■ These imaging techniques involve the administration of radionuclides (radiopharmaceuticals).

■ The emitted radiation is then measured, usually using a gamma camera.

■ Nuclear imaging is more concerned with the imaging of function, rather than structure, so the spatial resolution is lower than that of CT or MRI. It can identify abnormalities such as metastases by their abnormal metabolism compared to normal tissue.

■ Nuclear imaging can be used to investigate a number of systems, including endocrine (e.g. sestamibi imaging), cardiac (multiple-gated acquisition [MUGA] imaging and myocardial perfusion actinography), bone (bone scintigraphy and dual energy X-ray absorptiometry [DEXA]) and renal (mer-

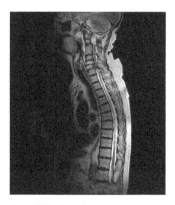

Figure 15.36: Cervical spine compression

captoacetyltriglycine [MAG3], diethylene triamine pentaacetic acid [DTPA] and dimercaptosuccinic acid [DMSA]).

■ Pregnancy is a contraindication to nuclear imaging, due to a risk of foetal damage (as for X-ray).

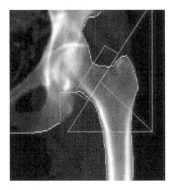

Figure 15.38: DEXA scan

Respiratory

V/Q imaging

■ Ventilation/perfusion lung imaging is accurate and non-invasive.

■ Ventilation and perfusion are matched in healthy individuals.

■ In pulmonary embolic disease, segmental reduction in perfusion occurs with maintenance of normal ventilation.

■ This leads to the mismatch of perfusion and ventilation in broncho-pulmonary segments.

■ In parenchymal lung disease matched ventilation and perfusion defects occur. In acute infection the ventilation defect may exceed the perfusion defect.

■ The primary indication is investigation of probability of pulmonary emboli (in patients with normal chest X-rays).

■ If patients have abnormal chest X-rays, a spiral CT is the preferred next investigation.

■ Results usually stratify risk as low, intermediate or high-probability of an embolus.

Bone scintigraphy (bone imaging)

Technetium-99m bone imaging

■ This is used to evaluate the distribution of active bone formation in the body.

■ It can be performed as a multi-phase study (blood flow, immediate and delayed imaging phases) and used to identify areas of abnormal bone metabolic activity.

■ When administered (intravenously), most of the technetium progressively accumulates in bone. The remainder is excreted in urine.

■ Increased uptake (is seen in immature and metabolically active bone (e.g. 'hot' sites of increased osteoblastic activity with new bone formation, such as at epiphyseal plates).

■ This investigation therefore provides a more functional assessment of bone.

■ Common indications include: neoplastic disease (looking for primary bone tumours and bone metastases), looking for avascular necrosis, occult and stress fractures, osteomyelitis, arthritides, bone infarct and reflex sympathetic dystrophy.

Cardiac

Multiple-gated acquisition (MUGA) imaging

■ Used to evaluate cardiac function, by enabling visualisation of myocardial contraction.

■ Utilises a combination of stannous ions and technetium-99m to label red blood cells.

■ The patient's heart beat is used to 'gate' the acquisition.

■ A series of images (usually 16) are produced for each stage of the cardiac cycle.

■ The ejection fraction is one of several parameters that can be determined.

Myocardial perfusion scintigraphy and stress tests

■ This single photon emission computed tomography (SPECT) procedure is used to investigate cardiac pathologies that affect the myocardium, including coronary artery disease and hypertrophic cardiomyopathy.

■ Thallium-201 and technetium-99m (Tc-99m) are most commonly used.

■ Left ventricular ejection fraction can be calculated.

■ This imaging is usually performed in conjunction with a cardiac stress test.

■ Stress tests utilise stressors (e.g. treadmill, bicycle, IV adenosine or IV dobutamine) and abnormalities reflect marked imbalances of relative blood flow to different portions of ventricular muscle tissue.

Endocrine

Thyroid and parathyroid imaging

■ Thyroid scintigraphy is used for assessing the functionality of thyroid lesions, by determining the relative uptake of Tc-99m, which is trapped by thyroid follicular cells.

■ ^{123}I-iodide is also used, and is both trapped and organified by thyroid follicular cells.

■ Common indications include the assessment of functionality of thyroid nodules and goitres, determining uptake prior to radio-iodine treatment and locating ectopic thyroid tissue.

NB: It is important that the patient does not have iodinated contrast prior to a radioactive iodine study.

Sestamibi

■ This is used to locate the parathyroid glands, usually for identifying hyperparathyroidism (parathyroid adenoma).

■ The Tc-99m sestamibi is taken up by both the thyroid and the parathyroids, with a greater rate of absorption in a hyperfunctioning parathyroid gland.

Neurological

SPECT

■ This uses Tc-99m attached to lipophilic hexamethylene propyleamine oxime (HMPAO), which can cross the blood–brain barrier.

■ Its purpose is to allow the level of cerebral blood flow and metabolism to be recorded.

■ This can be of use in the investigation of focal seizures (varying degrees of metabolism pre and post-ictally).

Positron emission tomography (PET)

■ This utilises a short-lived radioactive tracer isotope that decays, emitting a positron.

■ The tracer is attached to a metabolically active molecule, allowing it to accumulate in areas of elevated metabolic activity.

■ PET imaging is often used in conjunction with CT or MRI imaging, allowing the functional aspects of PET to be overlaid onto the anatomical detail of CT or MRI.

■ A tracer commonly used for PET imaging is 18-fluorodeoxyglucose (18-FDG), a glucose derivative. The tracer is administered intravenously, and the region of interest is subsequently imaged. 18-FDG decays, emitting protons. Collision of this proton with an electron results in two photons that are sent in opposite directions – the scanner detects these.

Uses

Uses include the following.

■ Oncology: for imaging tumours and locating metastasis. The differential glucose metabolism between the cancerous and normal tissue (i.e. the higher metabolic activity of the tumour) allows it to be localised better with this 'functional' imaging than with CT or MRI.

■ Neurology: for determining brain function in conditions such as Parkinson's disease and epilepsy, particularly in research settings.

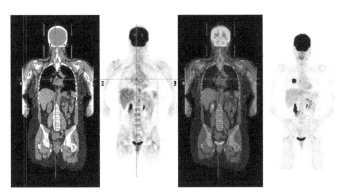

Figure 15.39: PET scan

Renal

Dimercaptosuccinic acid (DMSA) cortical scintigraphy

■ Tc-99m DMSA is injected IV. It is bound to the proximal tubules and provides information on relative (or differential) function of each kidney showing areas of scarring.

■ Indications include detection of renal parenchymal abnormalities (particularly scarring), assessment of renal function and subsequent scarring in vesico-ureteric reflux nephropathy and post

urinary tract infection (UTI) and the detection of congenital abnormalities, e.g. horseshoe, or ectopic kidneys. SPECT DMSA imaging can provide improved resolution.

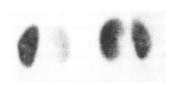

Figure 15.40: DMSA

Diethylene triamine pentaacetic acid (DTPA)

■ This uses Tc-99m. It allows dynamic imaging of renal function.

■ As the contrast agent is filtered by glomerulus and then rapidly excreted via the kidney, DTPA can be used for calculating glomerular filtration rate (GFR).

■ It provides renograms in three phases: vascular, accumulation within the kidney and excretion.

■ It is used to assess obstruction and reflux in children and to monitor graft function post-transplantation. Indications include the investigation of obstruction and renovascular disease, and the assessment of renal perfusion and bladder function.

■ A micturating cystogram (MCUG) is also used to follow-up vesico-ureteric reflux.

Mercaptoacetyltriglycine (MAG3)

■ MAG is a compound chelated with Tc-99m.

■ Radiolabelled MAG3 has a similar excretion pattern to DTPA and hippuran imaging, but provides better image definition especially in impaired renal function.

■ It can therefore provide both anatomical and functional information, and is the preferred technique in children.

Contrast studies

■ Contrast studies use radio-opaque substances to highlight the region of interest on other forms of radiological imaging (e.g. X-ray).

■ Different types of contrast agent are available:

• barium sulphate is commonly used for gastrointestinal (GI) tract studies

• iodine – in either an organic (non-ionic) or ionic compound form – is another commonly used agent. The organic form has fewer side effects and is water-soluble (it is more commonly used these days)

• gadolinium, a water-soluble agent, is commonly used for MRI.

■ Route of administration and side effects depend on the nature of the study and contrast agent used. A rare (but potentially serious) side effect associated with contrast agents is anaphylactoid reaction. Another important complication – particularly in patients with impaired renal function – is nephropathy.

■ Contraindications to the various agents also depend on the agent itself and the type of examination. For example, barium-based agents should not be used if there is suspected perforation or complete obstruction of the GI tract. If contrast imaging is indicated in these situations (or if there is patient allergy to barium), then gastrograffin should be used instead. This is a water-soluble agent. Iodine-based agents should not be used in patients taking metformin due to an increased risk of renal failure; this drug should be stopped prior to the study, and may be resumed approximately 48 h after the study (provided renal function is stable).

Biliary tract

Percutanenous trans-hepatic cholangiography (PTC)

■ In certain situations (e.g. tight strictures), visualisation of the biliary tract with endoscopic retrograde cholangio-pancreatography (ERCP) is not possible.

■ PTC involves injection of contrast agent through a fine needle inserted percutaneously into the intra-hepatic biliary tree to visualise dilated biliary ducts and identify the point of stricturing.

■ The dilated biliary system can be drained externally (via a percutaneously placed drainage tube) or internally (into the duodenum via percutaneously placed stent through the stricture site), through this access point.

Cardiovascular

Angiography

■ This involves the taking of serial contrast enhanced X-rays to visualise the lumen of blood vessels.

■ A catheter is introduced into a superficial access vessel, e.g. the common femoral artery. The catheter is then manipulated using a guide wire to the area and vessels of interest (e.g. coronary, carotid, visceral, renal, iliac, subclavian arteries). Contrast agent is injected via the catheter into the vessel, e.g. the renal artery, and images taken to show the vascular pattern and identify abnormalities, e.g. stenoses, fistulas.

■ The coronary vessels are commonly visualised, with the ability to dilate vessel stenoses using catheter-mounted balloons (angioplasty) or by inserting metallic stents.

■ Vessel haemorrhage can be treated by identifying the bleeding vessel by angiography and placing embolic material (e.g. coils, particles, glue) local to the bleeding point through the catheter.

Gastrointestinal

In a normal bowel, barium fills the lumen uniformly. Pathology can be detected by non-uniform filling and delays in transit.

Barium swallow

■ This single contrast study is used to assess the functional and anatomical properties of the oesophagus.

■ Liquid barium contrast is swallowed and radiographs are taken during the oesophageal transit phase.

■ Any regurgitation of gastric contents can be subsequently assessed by taking further images with the patient in a head-down position.

■ For the investigation of dysphagia, bread soaked in barium can be used.

■ Indications for a barium swallow include dysphagia, odynophagia, gastro-oesophageal reflux and the investigation of several oesophageal disorders, e.g. achalasia.

Water-soluble swallow

■ A water-soluble agent is used instead of barium as the contrast agent in cases of oesophageal tear or rupture. In these situations barium can cause a chemical mediastinitis.

Barium meal

■ This double-contrast study consists of a series of upper gastrointestinal tract X-rays taken after ingestion of barium sulphate containing a contrast medium accompanied by a two-part gas-producing agent (used to cause visceral distension).

■ By following the ingestion and flow down the oesophagus, stomach and duodenum, the structure and motility of the upper GI tract can be investigated.

■ By allowing the contrast agent to evenly cover the inner stomach lining, and taking X-ray images from different angles, it is possible to assess the stomach mucosa looking for abnormalities such as ulcers.

- Indications for a barium meal include hiatus hernia, gastric/duodenal malignancy, peptic ulcer disease.

Small bowel follow-through
- Used to investigate the small bowel.
- After the contrast agent (usually a barium sulphate compound) is orally administered, serial X-rays are taken at delayed time intervals to allow the contrast to travel through the small bowel.
- The examination usually takes about 2–3 h.
- Structures visualised include the duodenum, jejunum and ileum.
- The small bowel is characterised by plicae circulares (valvulae conniventes).
- There is a progressive decrease in size of the bowel lumen from jejunum to ileum, with a smoother lumen in the ileum.
- Indications for a small bowel follow-through include Crohn's disease, malabsorption, fistulae, GI bleeds, incomplete small bowel obstruction and suspected tumours.

Barium enema
- This examines the lower gastrointestinal tract (anus, rectum, colon and appendix).
- This is usually a double-contrast examination (barium sulphate and air). The liquid barium containing contrast agent is inserted per rectally via a tube as an enema. This is followed by the per-rectal insufflation of air to distend the bowel for better visualisation of the bowel mucosa. Buscopan is often given intravenously to prevent bowel spasm.

- Some investigative uses include assessing for inflammatory bowel disease (strictures, fistulae), polyps, tumours and diverticulosis.

Water-soluble (or gastrograffin) enema
- If perforation is suspected, a water-soluble contrast is used to avoid the serious risks of barium leaks into the peritoneal cavity, which is associated with a high mortality (>50%).
- This is also used in suspected large bowel obstruction to help determine the level of obstruction, as well as to differentiate a sigmoid volvulus from a sigmoid pseudo-obstruction.

Renal

IVU/IVP
- Intravenous urography (IVU) is used to investigate suspected urinary tract obstruction.
- Also known as IV pyelography (IVP), this involves taking serial KUB (kidney, ureter, bladder) X-rays at timed intervals after the administration of an IV contrast medium (typically iodinated contrast agent).
- Image-intensified fluoroscopy can also allow real-time studies of urinary tract flow. Post-voiding films can also demonstrate any residual urine in the bladder.
- IVU allows visualisation of the renal calyces and papillae, and can also be useful in the diagnosis of intrinsic renal pathology, such as papillary necrosis or medullary sponge kidney.
- Radiolucent stones, clots and tumours can be seen, as well as abnor-

malities in the ureteric wall, e.g. hydronephrosis, strictures and external pathological compression.

■ Note that these techniques are increasingly being replaced by computed tomography urogram (CTU) for the investigation of renal calculi.

Antegrade pyelography

■ This involves percutaneous injection of contrast directly into the renal pelvis followed by serial X-ray imaging.

■ It can show sites of obstruction and also allows relief of the obstruction via the nephrostomy.

Retrograde pyelography

■ A small ureteric catheter is placed in the renal pelvis via a cystoscope. Contrast agent is injected via the catheter during radiographic screening to look for filling defects in the renal pelvis or ureter. It is used to detect lower urinary tract abnormalities and to look for multifocal disease in transitional cell carcinoma.

Cystography

■ Contrast agent is instilled directly into the bladder via a transurethral or suprapubic catheter. Allows the investigation of bladder disease.

Voiding cystourethrography

■ Serial X-rays of the bladder and urethra are taken during micturition, allowing the detection of conditions such as vesico-ureteric reflux.

Bone density imaging

DEXA (Dual energy X-ray absorptiometry)

■ The gold standard for measuring bone mineral density and, subsequently, assessing fracture risk.

■ This involves the use of two X-ray beams of different intensities. The bone mineral density is then calculated by subtracting the soft-tissue signal from the resulting images.

■ It is commonly used in the diagnosis of osteoporosis (lumbar spine and femoral neck are normally assessed).

■ Risks and contraindications are similar as for X-rays.

■ Results are quoted as a T-score or a Z-score (allows osteoporotic fracture risk stratification by considering an individual's relative age and risk factors).

■ **T-scores:** number of standard deviations (SD) from the young adult mean:
• normal: T- score > -1 (i.e. within 1 SD of the young adult mean)
• osteopaenia: T-score > -1 to -2.5 (i.e. between 1 and 2.5 SD below the young adult mean)
• osteoporosis: T-score < -2.5 (i.e. 2.5 SD below the young adult mean).

■ **Z-scores:** number of SD from the age-related mean. Does not allow diagnosis of osteoporosis (requires T-score); however, it is useful in age-related risk stratification.

Radiation doses

NB: Chest X-ray = 2 × background radiation dose.

Equivalent numbers of chest X-rays

Investigation	Radiation dose (mSv)	Number of CXR
Plain X-rays		
Chest	0.02	1
Abdomen	1.5	75
Cervical spine	0.1	5
Hip	0.3	15
Lumbar spine	2.4	120
Extremities, e.g. knee	0.01	0.5
IVU	1.6	80
Fluoroscopy/Screening studies		
Barium swallow	2	100
Barium meal	6	300
Barium follow-through	5	250
CT studies		
CT chest	8	400
CT abdomen	10	500
CT head	2	100
CT cervical spine	10	500
Nuclear medicine studies		
Bone scintigram	3.8	190
Lung V/Q	1.2	60
Myocardial perfusion	12	600
Thyroid	1	50

Adapted from Donald, A & Stein, M. (2006) The hands-on guide for junior doctors. Blackwell Publishing, Oxford.

Presenting imaging findings

■ It may sound obvious, but speak slowly and clearly. Try not to rush through the presentation, even though you can see an obvious abnormality. There may be more than meets the eye, so make sure you stick to your set structure for working through the images.

■ Always present the background first (i.e. patient details, etc.).

■ Look at the whole image, not just what you think may be wrong; remember to keep looking for abnormalities on the film while slowly presenting the background – this can also buy you more time.

■ If there is an obvious abnormality, it may be helpful to state this at the outset.

■ Then, make sure you work through a set structure through the rest of the film.

■ The key is practice, practice, practice.

Tips on making radiology requests

■ Be polite and fill in the request form in adequate detail.

■ Know why you want the investigation ('my consultant said so' probably does not count as an indication). Think about what you might expect to see, why the particular imaging modality you have requested is best, and how you might manage what you find.

■ It is likely that you will have several different requests to make. Prioritise the requests on clinical urgency. If you are not sure which is more urgent, ask one of your seniors.

■ Know the patient's past medical history. Fifteen minutes reading through the patient's notes will help you with all aspects of that patient's management and will give you an insight into any other problems that the patient may not yet have told you about. For a patient with a complex investigative history, it may be of use to take the patient's notes to the radiologist for them to review for clarification.

■ Know the patient's imaging history. This is easily gleaned from the radiology reports and many hospitals have computerised radiology information systems. You may find that the patient has already had the test that you are asking for.

■ Certain imaging may be contraindicated in certain situations, e.g. in suspected perforation, gastrograffin rather than barium should be used. Know possible contraindications to the test you are requesting. Other potential problems are pregnancy (for imaging involving radiation), difficulty lying still or claustrophobia (for CT/MRI), renal failure (for contrast-based imaging), metalwork (for MRI), etc. Always minimise radiation exposure.

■ When you make the request, let the radiology department know if the patient has any other problems or conditions that will affect the timing or type of imaging used, e.g. does the patient have methicillin-resistant *Staphylococcus aureus* (MRSA) infection or *Clostridium difficile* diarrhoea? Is the patient significantly obese and too heavy for the radiology equipment? The radiology department will have to use special precautions on occasion, and arrange the timing of investigations so as not to cross-contaminate patients.

■ Finally, look at previous imaging studies when interpreting the present image – serial images are often far more useful than isolated ones.

Chapter 16
PATIENT DATA

Introduction

This chapter contains practical tips on how to work with some of the commonly encountered documents and charts relevant to patient care. The key with all of these is to ensure that anything you document is clear and accurate. With observation charts, work through the data methodically – as with many things in medicine, developing a system will help ensure you do not omit important findings.

Topics covered
- Observation charts
- Specialised charts
- Intravenous fluid composition
- Documentation in clinical notes
- Pre-operative assessment

Observation charts

The observation or 'obs' charts found on every ward, contain basic patient data. These can include information about a number of parameters. Please note that, as for Chapter 1, all quoted reference ranges can vary between normal individuals and can be dependent on a number of criteria, including age, sex, race, etc. They are therefore guides only.

Variable	Normal value
Patient details (name/hospital number/DOB)	–
Pulse (heart rate, HR)	60–100 beats/min
Blood pressure (BP)	120/80 mmHg (age dependent)
Respiratory rate	12–20 breaths/min
Oxygen saturation	≈ 97% (on room air)
Temperature	36.5–37.5°C
Neurological observations (including pupil size, Glasgow Coma Scale [GCS] and 'Alert, Voice-response, Pain-response, Unresponsive' scale [AVPU])	GCS = 15/15 AVPU = 'A' (alert), 'V' (voice response), 'P' (pain response), 'U' (unresponsive). (See Chapter 7 for further details)
Urine output	Adults: ½–1 mL/kg/h
Weight	Variable
Body mass index (BMI)	20–25 kg/m²
Stool frequency/consistency	Variable

The hands-on guide to data interpretation. By S. Abraham, K. Kulkarni, R. Madhu and D. Provan.
Published 2010 by Blackwell Publishing Ltd.

These observations are recorded at set frequencies, for example twice a day in more stable patients, or every 15 minutes in unstable patients who are at risk of a deteriorating clinical condition.

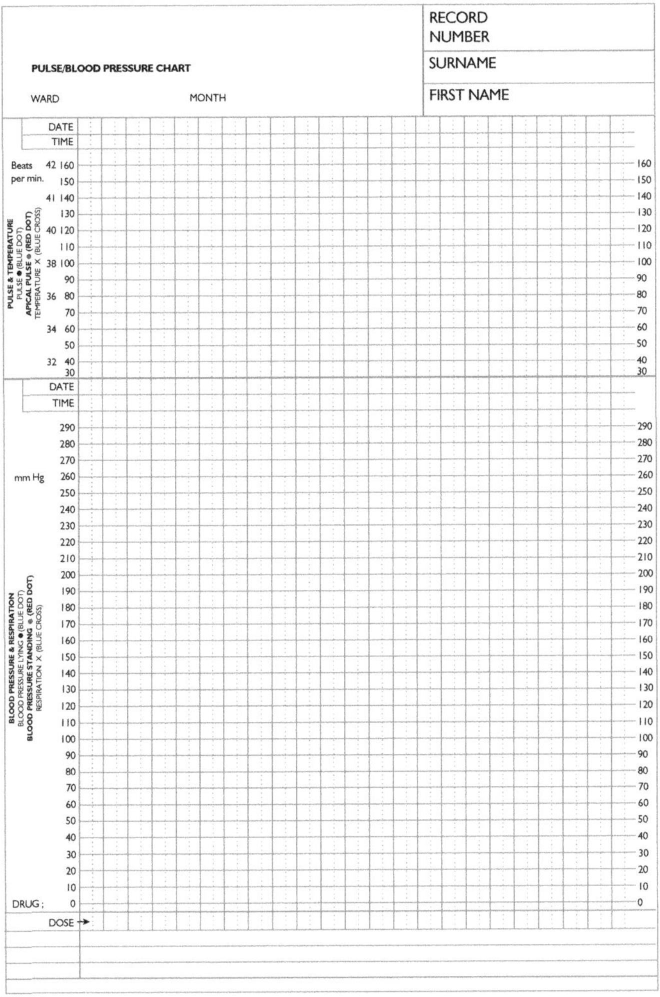

Figure 16.1: Patient observation chart

Specialised charts

■ There is a vast range of more specialised charts that can be used to record, observe or define various aspects of a patient's condition or management.

■ Remember that the **pattern** of the data over time is just as important as the numbers themselves. For example, one-off recordings of low BP may suggest a different pathology to a steadily falling BP.

■ We have included some examples of such charts below.

Drug charts
■ Allergies
■ Drugs to be administered
■ Dose
■ Start/stop date and time
■ Route and frequency of administration

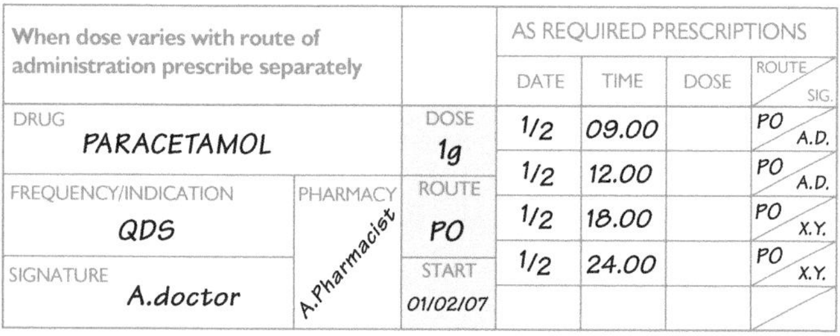

When dose varies with route of administration prescribe separately			AS REQUIRED PRESCRIPTIONS			
			DATE	TIME	DOSE	ROUTE / SIG.
DRUG PARACETAMOL		DOSE 1g	1/2	09.00		PO / A.D.
FREQUENCY/INDICATION QDS	PHARMACY A.Pharmacist	ROUTE PO	1/2	12.00		PO / A.D.
			1/2	18.00		PO / X.Y.
SIGNATURE A.doctor		START 01/02/07	1/2	24.00		PO / X.Y.

Figure 16.2: Drug prescription chart

Fluid balance/prescriptions charts
■ Record fluids and infusions to be administered, as well as:
• timeframe (e.g. over 8 h)
• route (e.g. IV)
• supplements (e.g. 20 mmol potassium chloride to a bag of normal saline).
■ Fluid balance charts record both inputs and outputs over a defined time period (e.g. 24 h) and play a vital role in

patient management. These charts include:
- inputs: oral, nasogastric (NG) and intravenous (IV) routes
- outputs: urine, vomit/aspirate and any other significant outputs (e.g. stoma, surgical drains).

■ Remember that inputs should equal outputs – while a 'normal' or healthy individual has a requirement of approximately 3 L per day (average-sized male), this requirement can increase/decrease depending on the situation; for example, if a patient has considerable fluid losses through a post-operative drain, these must be carefully replaced.

■ Other observations and measurements are also useful in guiding fluid replacement, including symptoms (thirst); clinical examination (decreased skin turgor, capillary refill time, blood pressure, concentrated urine); blood results (urea, creatinine).

Intensive care unit and anaesthetic charts

■ These are essentially more detailed versions of several other charts, integrating multiple areas, including clinical observations, fluid balance/prescription, drug prescriptions and blood results.

■ Anaesthetic charts are used pre/intra/post-operatively to record the patient's status. Like intensive care unit charts, data are recorded considerably more frequently than with standard 'ward' observation charts as changes in observations can occur more rapidly with these groups of patients

Peak-expiratory flow chart

■ As discussed in the respiratory chapter, serial measurements (i.e. trends over time) are more useful than isolated one-off measurements.

■ Patients should therefore keep a 'peak-flow diary' to record these, as such records will incorporate observations such as morning/evening variations.

Cardiovascular risk assessment curves

■ These charts are designed for estimating cardiovascular disease (CVD) risk (i.e. non-fatal myocardial infarction and stroke, coronary and stroke death, and new angina pectoris) in individuals who have not yet developed coronary heart disease (CHD) or other major atherosclerotic disease.

■ They are included here as an example of one of the many type of 'specialist' charts that are useful in patient management (the range is vast – from neonatal height/weight centile charts to prognostic curves for malignancies).

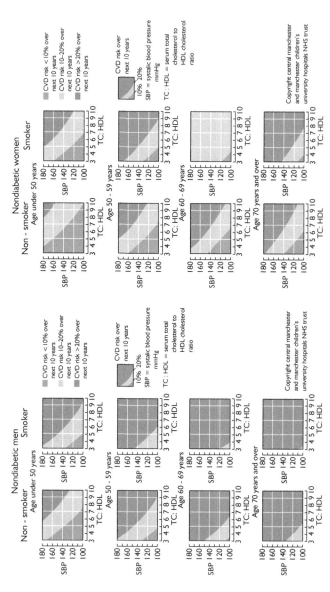

Figure 16.3: *Cardiovascular risk assessment charts. Source: Wood DA, Wray R, Poulter N, Williams, et al. (2005) JBS2: Joint British guidelines on prevention of cardiovascular disease in clinical practice. Heart* **91**(Suppl V): V1–52. www.bhsoc.org/Cardiovascular_Risk_Prediction_Chart.stm.

Intravenous fluid composition

Crystalloids

Fluid	mmol/L				Extras	pH
	Na⁺	K⁺	Ca²⁺	Cl⁻		
0.9% Normal saline	150	–	–	150	–	5.0
5% Dextrose	–	–	–	–	50 g dextrose (278 mmol/L glucose)	4.0
Dextrose saline (4%/0.18% respectively)	30	–	–	30	40 g dextrose (185 mmol/L glucose)	4.0
Hartmann's (Ringer's lactate)	131	5	2	111	29 mmol/L lactate	6.5
Gelofusine	154	5	6.25	120	40 g gelatin	7.4

Documentation in clinical notes

Medical records are legal documents. Writing clear notes is therefore of vital importance. The aim of your entry should be to convey the problems, the assessment and the management plan in a concise manner to allow colleagues (medical and other healthcare professionals, e.g. nurse, physiotherapist, etc.) to understand and continue the patient's care. In some hospitals there are separate sets of records for doctors' notes and other healthcare professionals' notes – make sure you read both sets so you get an understanding of the big picture. Always remember to document not only medical problems, but also other management issues, such as conversations with patients and their families or discussions you have with other people regarding the patient and their care.

Essentials

■ Clear handwriting, with a black pen (a ballpoint pen rather than ink): notes may need to be photocopied.

■ Date and time every entry (24-h clock format).

■ Signature: include your name, designation (e.g. F1 House Officer) and bleep number.

■ Avoid the use of abbreviations as these can lead to confusion. However, there are some established abbreviations that are in common use, e.g. 1/7 (1 day), etc.

■ Be very clear with units when documenting drug doses.

■ If you are documenting notes as part of a senior's ward round, document the name of your senior colleague and their designation clearly at the top of the entry. You should still sign the entry with your own details at the end.

■ Make sure the patient's details (ideally a patient information sticky label with name, date of birth and hospital number) are at the top of every page of the notes.

■ Make sure the notes are filed in the correct order and that there are a couple of blank history sheets at the end. A few extra seconds spent re-arranging will pay dividends when you are struggling to write in lots of sets of notes on a busy ward round.

■ If you make an error, strike through the error with a single line (so the original text is still visible). Write the word 'error' above the mistake and always sign, time and date the crossed out text. For example:

(error, Dr D Jones 14.00, 14/01/08)
Pain in ~~left~~ right iliac fossa

What should be included?

The 'SOAP' strategy is a good one to follow.

Subjective

This should contain subjective observations. These are the comments the patient/another observer expresses to you. Such observations include the patient's descriptions of their symptoms (e.g. 'patient is experiencing a dull pain in their left calf'), as well as other non-medical issues (e.g. 'patient is concerned about what will happen when they start walking').

Objective

This is an objective observation of the problem. These include symptoms/signs that can actually be measured or otherwise objectively experienced, e.g. vital signs (such as temperature or

pulse), descriptions of the problem (e.g. a 4-cm fluctuant swelling above the left nipple, etc.), as well as the results of diagnostic investigations (e.g. Full blood count: Hb 8.2 g/dL, CXR: left lower zone consolidation) and examination findings.

Examination findings are often labelled 'O/E' or 'on examination'. You should then proceed to document the relevant vital signs (observations), your general findings (e.g. visibly jaundiced, clubbing) and your specific system-based findings.

Assessment

This is your diagnosis or conclusion based on the above findings. In cases where several potential diagnosis or problems exist, it can be useful to make a clear problem list. For example:

Problems

1 Shortness of breath (secondary to left lower zone pneumonia).

2 Dysuria (secondary to confirmed urinary tract infection).

Plan

This is your management plan. It should include any investigations ordered (e.g. laboratory, radiological), drugs prescribed (with doses and duration of treatment), procedures required (e.g. abdominal ascitic paracentesis required), referrals (to a specialist or another professional, e.g. a social worker referral) and other general discharge related information (e.g. patient medically fit for discharge – awaiting bed in community hospital) as well as information given to the patient and follow-up details (Dr Murphy outpatient clinic appointment booked in 2/52).

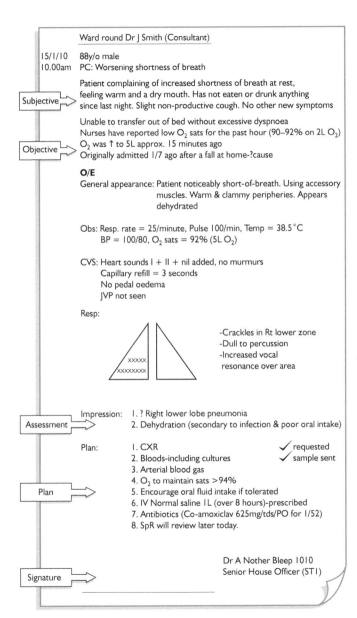

Ward round Dr J Smith (Consultant)

15/1/10
10.00am

88y/o male
PC: Worsening shortness of breath

Subjective

Patient complaining of increased shortness of breath at rest,
feeling warm and a dry mouth. Has not eaten or drunk anything
since last night. Slight non-productive cough. No other new symptoms

Objective

Unable to transfer out of bed without excessive dyspnoea
Nurses have reported low O_2 sats for the past hour (90–92% on 2L O_2)
O_2 was ↑ to 5L approx. 15 minutes ago
Originally admitted 1/7 ago after a fall at home-?cause

O/E

General appearance: Patient noticeably short-of-breath. Using accessory
muscles. Warm & clammy peripheries. Appears
dehydrated

Obs: Resp. rate = 25/minute, Pulse 100/min, Temp = 38.5 °C
BP = 100/80, O_2 sats = 92% (5L O_2)

CVS: Heart sounds I + II + nil added, no murmurs
Capillary refill = 3 seconds
No pedal oedema
JVP not seen

Resp:

xxxxx
xxxxxxxx

-Crackles in Rt lower zone
-Dull to percussion
-Increased vocal
 resonance over area

Assessment

Impression: 1. ? Right lower lobe pneumonia
              2. Dehydration (secondary to infection & poor oral intake)

Plan

Plan: 1. CXR   ✓ requested
        2. Bloods-including cultures   ✓ sample sent
        3. Arterial blood gas
        4. O_2 to maintain sats >94%
        5. Encourage oral fluid intake if tolerated
        6. IV Normal saline 1L (over 8 hours)-prescribed
        7. Antibiotics (Co-amoxiclav 625mg/tds/PO for 1/52)
        8. SpR will review later today.

Signature

Dr A Nother Bleep 1010
Senior House Officer (ST1)

Figure 16.4: Sample entry in medical notes

Emergencies

If you are asked to review a patient in an emergency setting (e.g. a patient with severe chest pain), a useful strategy to use for your 'assessment' can be to use the 'ABC' approach. For example:

A Airway clear, patient maintaining own airway, sitting upright.

B Breathing spontaneously, using accessory muscles
Respiratory rate = 25/min
O_2 sats = 95% (on 100% O_2 through re-breather mask)
No peripheral cyanosis

C Patient appears well hydrated
BP = 130/80, pulse = 100/min
Capillary refill = 3 s
Heart sounds I + II + no added sounds + no murmurs
ECG: sinus tachycardia

Documentation of clinical examination

■ When documenting your clinical examination findings in the notes, it can be helpful to draw an appropriate diagram so that you can note the exact site at which any symptoms or signs are present.

■ As with the charts discussed above, remember that the notes are a legal document. Ensure your writing is legible, and sign, date and cross through any errors with a single, clear line.

■ Always avoid abbreviations – they are unclear and can be misleading.

■ The following diagrams are commonly used.

Respiratory

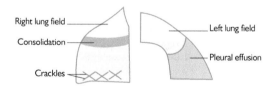

Right lung field
Consolidation
Crackles
Left lung field
Pleural effusion

Figure 16.5: Lung fields

Gastrointestinal

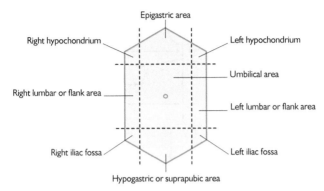

Figure 16.6: Regions of the abdomen

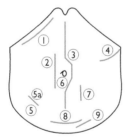

1. Kocher's (e.g. cholecystectomy). If extended along costal margin = subcostal
2. Right paramedian (laparotomy)
3. Midline laparotomy (commonest site for laparotomy)
4. Nephrectomy/loin (goes across to back, e.g. renal surgery)
5. Gridiron (appendicectomy)
5a. Lanz (appendicectomy)
6. Laparoscopic port insertion (e.g. for cholecystectomy/appendicectomy/colectomies)
7. Left paramedian (laparotomy, e.g. anterior rectal resection)
8. Transverse suprapubic/Pfannenstiel (hysterectomy/other pelvic surgery)
9. Inguinal hernia repair

Figure 16.7: Abdominal surgical incisions

Vascular

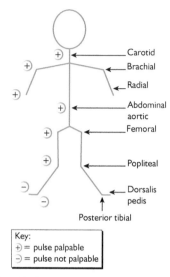

Key:
⊕ = pulse palpable
⊖ = pulse not palpable

Figure 16.8: Peripheral arterial pulses

Neurological

A similar diagram to the one above can be used for documenting the presence of peripheral reflexes.

Pre-operative assessment

■ This is an integral part of ensuring patient safety before, during and after surgery.

■ By ensuring that the patient's baseline status is optimised, any risks attributable to the stress placed on the body by surgery can be minimised.

■ Pre-operative assessment, commonly performed in the outpatient or clinic setting, includes several elements:

• clinical history and examination
• baseline observations
• baseline investigations: depending on the patient, their age/history and the nature of the procedure, a number of investigations can be performed, including:

– urinalysis (including pregnancy testing)

– blood (including full blood count, urea and electrolytes, liver function, clotting function, cross match, group and save, sickle cell testing)

– electrocardiogram (ECG)

– more specialised tests such as imaging, spirometry, etc.

– in addition, the anaesthetist will conduct an examination of the airway to evaluate the ease of intubation.

The American Society of Anaesthesiologists' (ASA) grading

■ The decision as to which pre-operative investigations are required, are based on ASA Grade and level of surgery or specialty.

■ There are special cases (e.g. neurosurgery, cardiac surgery).

■ Co-morbidities (e.g. cerebrovascular/respiratory/renal disease) should also be considered.

■ For example, for 'Grade 1' surgery (note that the thresholds vary between departments):

• fit and healthy children (<16 years), who are ASA Grade 1 require no pre-operative testing
• ASA grade 1 adults; consider ECG if >40 years and U&E if >60years
• ASA Grade 2 adults with cardiovascular disease require an ECG. Also consider:
– CXR if >40 years
– FBC any age
– U&E any age
– urinalysis.

Grade	Status	Absolute mortality (%)
I	A normal healthy patient. The process for which the operation is being performed is localised and causes no systemic upset	0.1
II	Mild systemic disease. All patients older than 80 years are put in this category	0.2
III	Severe systemic disease. This from any cause that imposes a definite functional limitation on their activity, e.g. chronic obstructive pulmonary disease	1.8
IV	Incapacitating systemic disease which is a constant threat to life	7.8
V	A moribund patient unlikely to survive 24h with or without surgery	9.4

Grading of surgical procedures by severity

The table below provides examples of different procedures that fall under the four grades of surgical risk.

Grade 1	■ Drainage of the middle ear ■ Minor dental surgery (e.g. tooth extraction)
Grade 2	■ Electroconvulsive therapy (ECT) ■ Partial breast excision ■ Extraction of lens ■ Haemorrhoid procedures
Grade 3	■ Bladder surgery (open) ■ Hysterectomy ■ Thyroidectomy ■ Total mastectomy
Grade 4	■ Major bowel surgery (e.g. colectomy) ■ Renal transplant ■ Total hip replacement

Index

Printed and bound by CPI Group (UK) Ltd, Croydon, CR0 4YY

27/10/2024

14580386-0001